Diagnostic Ultrasound

Diagnostic Ultrasound
Physical Principles and Exercises

Frederick W. Kremkau, Ph.D.

Research Assistant Professor of Medicine
Bowman Gray School of Medicine
Wake Forest University
Winston-Salem, North Carolina

Grune & Stratton
A Subsidiary of Harcourt Brace Jovanovich, Publishers
New York   London   Toronto   Sydney   San Francisco

Library of Congress Cataloging in Publication Data
Kremkau, Frederick W.
   Diagnostic ultrasound.

   Includes bibliographical references and index.
   1. Diagnosis, Ultrasonic. 2. Diagnosis,
Ultrasonic—Examinations, questions, etc.   I. Title.
RC78.7.U4K74   616.07'544   79-28250
ISBN 0-8089-1233-X

Grune & Stratton, Inc.
111 Fifth Avenue
New York, New York 10003

Distributed in the United Kingdom by
Academic Press, Inc. (London) Ltd.
24/28 Oval Road, London NW 1

Library of Congress Catalog Number 79-28250
International Standard Book Number 0-8089-1233-X
Printed in the United States of America

To Lil and Jonathan

Contents

Acknowledgments xi
Preface xiii

Chapter 1. Introduction   1
      1.1 Motivation
      1.2 The Big Picture
Chapter 2. Ultrasound   5
      2.1 Introduction
      2.2 Waves and Sound
      2.3 Pulsed Ultrasound
      2.4 Amplitude and Intensity
      2.5 Attenuation and Impedance
      2.6 Review
Chapter 3. Reflection, Scattering, Refraction, and Doppler Effect   29
      3.1 Introduction
      3.2 Normal Incidence and Scattering
      3.3 Oblique Incidence and Refraction
      3.4 Doppler Effect
      3.5 Attenuation and Reflection Combined
      3.6 Range Equation and Multiple Reflections
      3.7 Longitudinal Resolution and Useful Frequency Range
      3.8 Review
Chapter 4. Transducers and Sound Beams   54
      4.1 Introduction
      4.2 Transducers

4.3 Sound Beams
4.4 Lateral Resolution and Focusing
4.5 Arrays
4.6 Review

Chapter 5. Instrumentation   79
5.1 Introduction
5.2 Imaging System
5.3 Receiver
5.4 Display
5.5 Real Time
5.6 Doppler System
5.7 Artifacts
5.8 Review

Chapter 6. Performance Measurements   120
6.1 Introduction
6.2 Imaging Performance
6.3 Acoustic Output
6.4 Beam Profile
6.5 Review

Chapter 7. Bioeffects and Safety   132
7.1 Introduction
7.2 Bioeffects
7.3 Safety
7.4 Review

Chapter 8. Summary   140

Glossary   146

Answers to Exercises in the Text   154

Appendix 1. Equations List   167

Appendix 2. Physics Concepts   170
A2.1 Introduction
A2.2 Force and Pressure
A2.3 Motion
A2.4 Mass, Density, and Stiffness
A2.5 Law of Motion
A2.6 Work, Energy, and Power

Appendix 3. Algebra and Trigonometry   175
A3.1 Introduction
A3.2 Algebra
A3.3 Trigonometry

Appendix 4. Logarithms and Decibels   184
A4.1 Logarithms
A4.2 Decibels

Appendix 5. Units   189
    A5.1 Introduction
    A5.2 Tabulation
    A5.3 Manipulation
Appendix 6. Common Misconceptions   196
Answers to Exercises in the Appendixes   199
References   202
Index   205

Acknowledgments

The author gratefully acknowledges the assistance of the following persons: W. O'Brien, for critical review of the entire manuscript; L. Avecilla, R. Barnes, B. Bartley, E. Blackwell, P. Carson, C. Cole-Beuglet, L. Frizzell, S. Hagen-Ansert, R. Hileman, J. Korfhagen, R. Meyer, J. Nanasi, N. Nanda, P. Nuss, W. Nyborg, W. Riley, and A. Ring, for text review and criticism; J. Roselli, for artwork; R. Sturges, for typing; F. Yates, for proofreading; and J. Martin, for Center for Medical Ultrasound support.

Preface

This text is for sonographers and physicians who need basic knowledge of the acoustics and instrumentation of diagnostic ultrasound. Its purpose is to explain how diagnostic ultrasound works; it does not describe how to perform diagnostic examinations or interpret the results, except to point out artifact possibilities. It has been developed during the teaching of more than 300 students in 12 postgraduate courses on the subject. Little background in physics and mathematics is assumed. Help in these areas is available in Appendixes 2 through 5, which may be studied before beginning Chapter 1. More than 450 exercises are provided to check progress, strengthen concepts, and provide practice for registry and specialty boards examinations. Answers are given near the back of the book. Exercises in Sections 2.6, 3.8, 4.6, 5.8, 6.5, 7.4, and Chapter 8 may be used as pretests to determine knowledge in specific subject areas. Terms defined in the Glossary are boldface when first mentioned in the text.

Chapter 1

Introduction

There are five reasons for learning the material in this book:

1. to learn how diagnostic **ultrasound** works
2. to become aware of artifact possibilities
3. to pass the ultrasound physics portion of the registry and specialty boards examinations
4. to prepare for instrumentation performance measurement procedures
5. to become aware of safety and risk considerations

Ultrasound is useful in medical diagnosis primarily because it provides a method for visualizing internal body structures. The visualization method consists of two steps:

1. sending short **pulses** of ultrasound into the body
2. using **reflections** received from various tissues to produce an image of internal structures

The heart of the method is the interaction between ultrasound and tissues (Figure 1.1). The effects of the tissues on the ultrasound (**acoustic propagation properties**) are discussed in Chapters 2 and 3. This is the aspect of the interaction that is useful in diagnosis. The adjective

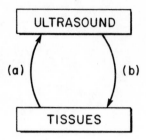

Figure 1.1. Interaction between ultrasound and tissues. (a) The effects of tissues on ultrasound are called the acoustic propagation properties of tisssues. They are what make ultrasound useful as a diagnostic tool. (b) The effects of ultrasound on tissues are called biological effects. They must be considered when discussing the safety of the diagnostic method.

acoustic refers to **sound. Propagation** means progression or travel. The effects of the ultrasound on tissues (biological effects) are considered in Chapter 7. Chapter 4 discusses how ultrasound is generated and received. The instrumentation that controls ultrasound generation and displays the received reflections is described in Chapter 5. Measurements for determining proper functioning of instrumentation are discussed in Chapter 6. The diagnostic ultrasound visualization method is described in Figure 1.2.

In addition to imaging, ultrasound provides a method for detecting motion and flow. The instruments that do this are described in Section 5.6.

Exercises

1.2.1. The diagnostic ultrasound visualization method has two parts:
  1. Sending short _____ of
  _____ into the body
  2. Using _____ received from various tissues to produce an _____ of internal structures

1.2.2. The heart of the diagnostic method is the interaction between _____ and _____ .

1.2.3. The effects of the tissues on ultrasound are called _____ propagation properties of tissues. They make ultrasound useful as a _____ tool.

1.2.4. The effects of ultrasound on tissues are called _____ effects.

1.2.5. Match the following to describe the steps of the diagnostic ultrasound visualization method:
  a. The operator controls the _____.   1. acoustic
  2. visual
  b. The instrumentation drives the _____.   3. transducer
  4. instrumentation

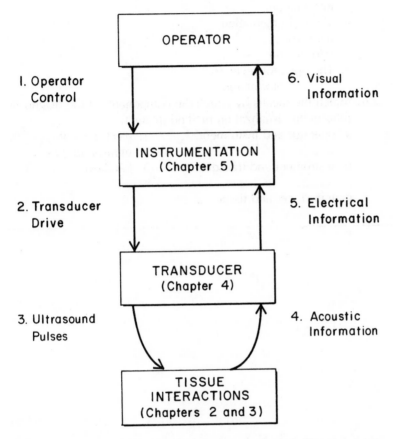

Figure 1.2. Diagnostic ultrasound visualization method. 1. The operator controls the operation of the instrumentation. 2. The instrumentation produces electrical voltages that drive the transducer. 3. The transducer produces ultrasound pulses that travel into the body and interact with the tissues. 4. The reflections generated in the tissues bring acoustic information to the transducer. 5. The transducer sends to the instrumentation electrical information corresponding to the received reflections. 6. The instrumentation converts the electrical information to visual form useful for medical diagnosis.

  c. The transducer
     produces ultrasound
     _____.
  d. The transducer
     receives _____
     information.
  e. The instrumentation
     receives _____
     information.
  f. The operator receives
     _____ information.

5. electrical
6. ultrasound pulses

1.2.6. Match the means by which the components of the diagnostic ultrasound visualization method interact:

  a. operator and instrument:
     _____

  b. instrument and transducer:
     _____

  c. transducer and tissue: _____

1. electrical voltages
2. ultrasound pulses
3. hand/eye

Chapter 2

Ultrasound

Ultrasound can provide information concerning internal body structures and motion. It is like the ordinary sound that we hear except that it has a **frequency** (discussed in the next section) higher than that to which the human hearing system can respond.

2.1 Introduction

Sound is a **wave.** A wave is a propagating (progressive or traveling) variation in quantities called **wave variables.** Waves carry **energy,*** not matter, from one place to another. Sound (Figure 2.1) is one particular type of wave. It is a propagating variation in quantities called **acoustic variables.** These acoustic variables include **pressure, density, temperature,** and **particle motion.** A **particle** is a small portion of the **medium** through which the sound is traveling. Unlike light waves and radio waves, sound requires a medium through which to travel. It cannot pass through a vacuum. Sound is a mechanical **longitudinal wave** in which back-and-forth particle motion is parallel to the direction of wave travel.

  Like all waves, sound is described by a few parameters. These are frequency, **period, wavelength, propagation speed, amplitude,** and **intensity.** Frequency, period, amplitude, and intensity are determined by

2.2 Waves and Sound

*This and other basic physics terms are discussed in Appendix 2.

Figure 2.1. Sound is traveling variations of acoustic variables (pressure, density, temperature, particle motion).

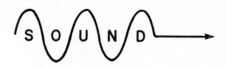

the sound source. Propagation speed is determined by the medium, and wavelength is determined by both the source and the medium.

Recall that sound is a traveling variation. Frequency tells how many complete variations **(cycles)** an acoustic variable goes through in a second. Take pressure as an example of an acoustic variable. Pressure may start at its normal value (atmospheric pressure), increase to a maximum value, return to normal, decrease to a minimum value, and return to normal. This describes a complete cycle of variation of pressure as an acoustic variable. As a sound wave travels past some point, this cycle is repeated over and over. The number of times that it occurs in 1 second is called the frequency (Figure 2.2).

Frequency units† include the **hertz (Hz)** and **megahertz (MHz)**. One hertz is one cycle per second or one complete variation per second. One megahertz is 1,000,000 Hz. Table A5.3 gives unit prefixes. Sound whose frequency is 20,000 Hz or higher is called ultrasound because it is beyond the frequency range of human hearing. Frequency will be important later when we consider image resolution and **depth of penetration.**

Period is the time that it takes for one cycle to occur (Figure 2.3). It is the reciprocal of frequency. Period units include seconds (s) and microseconds (μs). One microsecond is one-millionth of a second (0.000001 s). Period will be important when we consider **pulsed ultrasound** in Section 2.3. ‡

$$\text{period (s)} = \frac{1}{\text{frequency (Hz)}}$$

$$\text{period (}\mu\text{s)} = \frac{1}{\text{frequency (MHz)}}$$

Wavelength is the length of space over which one cycle occurs (Figure 2.4). Its units include meters (m) and millimeters (mm). One millimeter is one-thousandth of a meter (0.001 m). Wavelength will be important later when we consider image resolution.

†Units are discussed in Appendix 5.

‡For convenient reference, equations are compiled in Appendix 1.

6

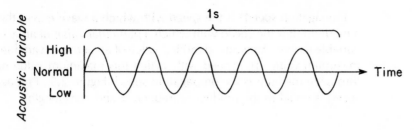

Figure 2.2. Frequency is the number of complete variations (cycles) that an acoustic variable goes through in 1 s. In this figure, five cycles occur each second; the frequency is five complete variations per second, or 5 Hz.

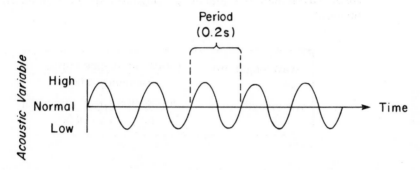

Figure 2.3. Period is the time it takes for one cycle to occur. In this figure, each cycle occurs in 0.2 s. The period is 0.2 s, and the frequency is the reciprocal of 0.2 s, or 5 Hz.

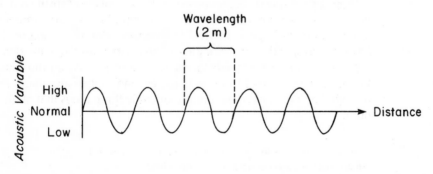

Figure 2.4. Wavelength is the length of space over which one cycle occurs. In this figure, each cycle covers 2 m. The wavelength is 2 m. This figure differs from Figures 2.2 and 2.3 in that the horizontal axis represents distance rather than time.

7

Propagation **speed*** is the speed with which a wave moves through a medium. It is the speed with which a *particular value* of an acoustic variable moves. An easily identified value of an acoustic variable is its maximum value. The speed with which this maximum value moves through a medium is the propagation speed (Figure 2.5). Propagation speed is equal to the product of frequency and wavelength.

> propagation speed (m/s) = frequency (Hz) x wavelength (m)
>
> propagation speed (mm/μs) =
> frequency (MHz) $\times$ wavelength (mm)

Also, wavelength is equal to propagation speed divided by frequency.†

> wavelength (m) = $\dfrac{\text{propagation speed (m/s)}}{\text{frequency (Hz)}}$
>
> wavelength (mm) = $\dfrac{\text{propagation speed (mm/}\mu\text{s)}}{\text{frequency (MHz)}}$

An example of the relationship among frequency, wavelength, and propagation speed may be seen by comparing Figures 2.2, 2.4, and 2.5 (see the legend for Figure 2.5). Propagation speed units include meters per second (m/s), kilometers per second (km/s), and millimeters per microsecond (mm/μs). One kilometer per second equals 1000 m/s. One millimeter per microsecond equals 1 km/s.

Propagation speed is determined by the density and **stiffness** (hardness) of the medium. Density is the concentration of matter (**mass** per unit volume). Stiffness is the resistance of a material to compression. Propagation speed increases if the stiffness is increased or if the density is *decreased* (a surprising fact for many students).‡ As an illustration, the propagation speed in brass is lower than that in aluminum even though the density of brass is approximately three times that of aluminum.

*Velocity is speed, with the direction of motion also specified.
†Basic algebra concepts are given in Appendix 3.
‡Common misconceptions are discussed in Appendix 6.

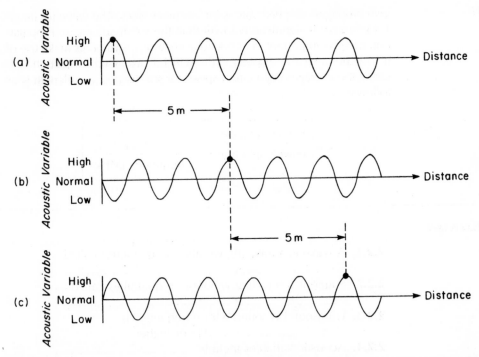

Figure 2.5. Propagation speed is the speed with which a particular value of an acoustic variable moves. The movement of a maximum (identified by the dot) is shown in this figure. Example (b) is 0.5 s after (a). Example (c) is 0.5 s after (b) and 1 s after (a). The maximum (dot) moves 5 m in 0.5 s and 10 m in 1 s. The propagation speed is 10 m/s. The frequency in Figure 2.2 (5 Hz) times the wavelength in Figure 2.4 (2 m) equals the propagation speed in this figure (10 m/s).

In general, propagation speeds through gases are low, through liquids are higher, and through solids are the highest. This *increasing* sequence is not caused by the increasing density (which produces a decreasing propagation speed) but by the increasing stiffness. This is because the stiffness differences are larger than the density differences. The average propagation speed in soft tissues is 1540 m/s, 1.54 km/s, or 1.54 mm/μs. In lung (which contains gas/air), the propagation speed is lower than in other soft tissues, generally in the range of 0.3–1.2 mm/μs.* The propagation speed in bone (a solid) is higher than that in soft tissue, generally in the range of 2–4 mm/μs.* Goss and associates[5]

---

*In Section 2.5 we will see that ultrasound does not penetrate lung or bone well, so that these differing propagation speeds are normally not of concern.

give propagation speed values for various tissues. The value for fat (~ 1.45 mm/μs) is significantly lower than the soft-tissue mean. Propagation speed is important to us because imaging instruments make use of it in generating the displays. This will be discussed in Section 5.4. Using the average propagation speed for soft tissues, wavelength is as follows:

$$\text{For soft tissues:}$$
$$\text{wavelength (mm)} = \frac{1.54}{\text{frequency (MHz)}}$$

Exercises

2.2.1. A wave is a traveling variation in quantities called
_____ _____ .

2.2.2. Sound is a traveling variation in quantities called
_____ _____ .

2.2.3. Ultrasound is sound whose frequency is
_____ Hz or higher.

2.2.4. Acoustic variables include _____ ,
_____ , _____ , and
_____ _____ .

2.2.5. Which of the following frequencies are in the ultrasound range? (More than one correct answer.)
a. 15 Hz
b. 15,000 Hz
c. 15 MHz
d. 30,000 Hz
e. 0.04 MHz

2.2.6. Which of the following are acoustic variables? (More than one correct answer.)
a. pressure
b. frequency
c. propagation speed
d. period
e. particle motion

2.2.7. Frequency is a measure of how many
_____ an acoustic variable goes through
in a second.

2.2.8. The unit for frequency is the _____ ,
which is abbreviated _____ .

2.2.9. Period is the _____ that it takes for one cycle to occur.

2.2.10. Period is the _____ of frequency.

2.2.11. Wavelength is the length of _____ over which one cycle occurs.

2.2.12. Propagation speed is the speed with which a _____ moves through a medium.

2.2.13. Wavelength is equal to _____ _____ divided by _____.

2.2.14. Propagation speed is determined by the _____ and _____ of a medium.

2.2.15. Propagation speed increases if
   a. density is increased
   b. density is decreased
   c. stiffness is increased
   d. a and c
   e. b and c

2.2.16. The average propagation speed in soft tissues is _____ m/s or _____ km/s or _____ mm/μs.

2.2.17. Propagation speed is determined by
   a. frequency
   b. amplitude
   c. wavelength
   d. period
   e. medium

2.2.18. Place the following in order of increasing sound propagation speed:
   a. gas
   b. solid
   c. liquid

2.2.19. The wavelength of 1-MHz ultrasound in soft tissues is _____ mm.

2.2.20. Wavelength in soft tissues _____ as frequency increases.

2.2.21. It takes _____ μs for ultrasound to travel 1.54 cm in soft tissue.

2.2.22. Propagation speed in bone is _____ than in soft tissues.

12

2.2.23. Sound travels fastest in
a. air
b. helium
c. water
d. iron
e. a vacuum

2.2.24. Solids have higher propagation speeds than liquids because they have higher
a. density
b. stiffness

2.2.25. The propagation speeds through mercury and fat are approximately the same, even though the density of mercury is approximately 15 times that of fat. This tells us that the stiffness of mercury must be much _____ than that of fat.

2.2.26. Sound is a _____ _____ wave.

2.2.27. If propagation speed is doubled (a different medium) and frequency is held constant, the wavelength is _____.

2.2.28. If wavelength in a given medium at a given frequency is 2 mm and the frequency is doubled, the wavelength becomes _____ mm.

2.2.29. If frequency in soft tissue is doubled, propagation speed is _____.

2.2.30. Waves carry _____ from one place to another.

2.2.31. From given values for propagation speed and frequency, which of the following can be calculated?
a. amplitude
b. period
c. wavelength
d. a and b
e. b and c

2.2.32. If two media have the same stiffness but different densities, the one with the higher density will have the higher propagation speed. True or false?

2.2.33. If two media have the same density but different stiffnesses, the one with the higher stiffness will have the higher propagation speed. True or false?

The terms discussed earlier (frequency, period, wavelength, and propagation speed) describe a **continuous wave (cw).** For diagnostic ultrasound imaging, continuous-wave sound is not commonly used. Instead, short pulses of sound are used. This is called pulsed ultrasound. It is produced by applying **electrical pulses** to the **transducer** (Chapter 4). Ultrasound pulses are described by some additional parameters that we have not yet introduced.

Pulse repetition frequency is the number of pulses occurring in a second (Figure 2.6). Its units include the hertz (Hz) and **kilohertz (kHz).** One kilohertz is 1000 Hz.

The **pulse repetition period** is the time from the beginning of one pulse to the beginning of the next (Figure 2.7). Its units include seconds (s) and milliseconds (ms). One millisecond is one-thousandth of a second (0.001 s). The pulse repetition period is the reciprocal of pulse repetition frequency.

$$\text{pulse repetition period (s)} = \frac{1}{\text{pulse repetition frequency (Hz)}}$$

$$\text{pulse repetition period (ms)} = \frac{1}{\text{pulse repetition frequency (kHz)}}$$

Pulse duration is the time that it takes for a pulse to occur (Figure 2.7). It is equal to the period times the number of cycles in the pulse. Its units include seconds (s) and microseconds (μs).

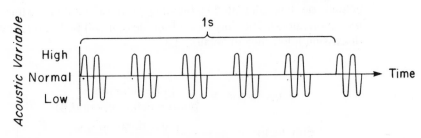

Figure 2.6. Pulse repetition frequency is the number of pulses occurring in 1 s. In this figure, five pulses (containing two cycles each) occur in 1 s; thus the pulse repetition frequency is 5 Hz.

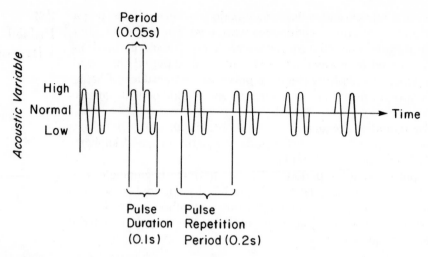

Figure 2.7. The pulse repetition period is the time from the beginning of one pulse to the beginning of the next. In this figure, the pulse repetition period is 0.2 s. Therefore the pulse repetition frequency is 5 Hz. Pulse duration is the time that it takes for one pulse to occur. It is equal to the period times the number of cycles in the pulse. In this figure, pulse duration is 0.1 s. Since two cycles occur in a 0.1-s pulse in this figure, the period is 0.05 s, and the frequency is 20 Hz. The duty factor is the fraction of time that the sound is actually on. It is pulse duration divided by pulse repetition period. The duty factor in this figure is 0.5.

$$
\begin{aligned}
\text{pulse duration (s)} \quad &= \text{number of cycles in the pulse} \times \\
&\quad \text{period (s)} \\[1ex]
\text{pulse duration } (\mu s) &= \text{number of cycles in the pulse} \times \\
&\quad \text{period } (\mu s) \\[1ex]
&= \frac{\text{number of cycles in the pulse}}{\text{frequency (MHz)}}
\end{aligned}
$$

Duty factor is the fraction of time that sound (in the form of pulses) is actually on. It is calculated by dividing the pulse duration by the pulse repetition period. The duty factor is unitless. It will be important when discussing intensities in Section 2.4.

$$
\begin{aligned}
\text{duty factor} &= \frac{\text{pulse duration (s)}}{\text{pulse repetition period (s)}} \\[2ex]
\text{duty factor} &= \frac{\text{pulse duration } (\mu s)}{\text{pulse repetition period (ms)} \times 1000}
\end{aligned}
$$

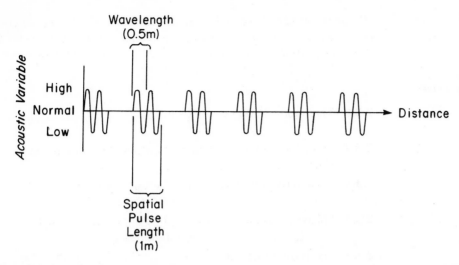

Figure 2.8. Spatial pulse length is the length of space over which a pulse occurs. It is equal to wavelength times the number of cycles in the pulse. In this figure, wavelength is 0.5 m, there are two cycles in each pulse, and spatial pulse length is 0.5 times 2, or 1 m. The frequency in Figure 2.7 (20 Hz) times the wavelength in this figure (0.5 m) equals the propagation speed (10 m/s). This figure differs from Figures 2.6 and 2.7 in that the horizontal axis represents distance rather than time.

Spatial pulse length is the length of space over which a pulse occurs (Figure 2.8). It is equal to the product of wavelength and the number of cycles in the pulse. Its units include meters (m) and millimeters (mm). It will be an important quantity when discussing **longitudinal resolution** in Section 3.7.

spatial pulse length (m)	=	number of cycles in the pulse × wavelength (m)
spatial pulse length (mm)	=	number of cycles in the pulse × wavelength (mm)
spatial pulse length (mm)	=	$\dfrac{\text{number of cycles in the pulse} \times \text{propagation speed (mm/}\mu\text{s)}}{\text{frequency (MHz)}}$
For soft tissues: spatial pulse length (mm)	=	$\dfrac{\text{number of cycles in the pulse} \times 1.54}{\text{frequency (MHz)}}$

Propagation speed for pulses is the same as that for continuous waves in a given medium. Frequency within pulses (as opposed to pulse repetition frequency) is the same as that for continuous waves.

Exercises

2.3.1. The abbreviation cw stands for _____ _____ .

2.3.2. Pulsed ultrasound is ultrasound in the form of repeated short _____ .

2.3.3. Pulse repetition frequency is the number of _____ occurring in 1 s.

2.3.4. Pulsed ultrasound is produced by applying electrical _____ to the transducer.

2.3.5. The pulse repetition _____ is the time from the beginning of one pulse to the beginning of the next.

2.3.6. The pulse repetition period is the _____ of pulse repetition frequency.

2.3.7. Pulse duration is the _____ for a pulse to occur.

2.3.8. Spatial pulse length is the _____ of _____ over which a pulse occurs.

2.3.9. _____ _____ is the fraction of time that pulsed ultrasound is actually on.

2.3.10. Pulse duration equals the number of the cycles in the pulse times _____ .

2.3.11. Spatial pulse length equals the number of cycles in the pulse times _____ .

2.3.12. The duty factor of continuous-wave sound is _____ .

2.3.13. If the wavelength is 2 mm, the spatial pulse length for a three-cycle pulse is _____ mm.

2.3.14. The spatial pulse length in soft tissue for a four-cycle pulse of frequency 3 MHz is _____ mm.

2.3.15. The pulse duration in soft tissue for a four-cycle pulse of frequency 3 MHz is _____ μs.

2.3.16. For a 1-kHz pulse repetition frequency, the pulse repetition period is _____ ms.

2.3.17. For Problems 2.3.15 and 2.3.16, the duty factor is _____ .

We have described the rate at which cycles occur in time (frequency), the time required for each cycle (period), the space over which a cycle occurs (wavelength), and the speed at which the cycles move (propagation speed). We shall now consider how great the variations are. This gives us some idea of the **strength** of the sound. Amplitude and intensity are the parameters that are relevant here.

Amplitude is the maximum variation that occurs in an acoustic variable. It is the maximum value minus the normal value (Figure 2.9). Amplitude is given in units appropriate for the acoustic variable considered.

Intensity is the **power** in a wave divided by the **beam area.** Power is

$$\text{intensity (W/cm}^2\text{)} = \frac{\text{power (W)}}{\text{beam area (cm}^2\text{)}}$$

discussed in Section A2.6. Power units include watts (W) and milliwatts (mW). **Sound beams** and beam area will be discussed in Section 4.3. Beam area units are centimeters squared (cm²). Intensity units include watts per centimeter squared (W/cm²) and others listed in Table A5.4. Intensity is an important parameter in describing the sound that is produced and received by diagnostic instrumentation (Chapter 5) and in discussing biological effects and safety (Chapter 7). It may be illustrated by analogy with sunlight incident on dry leaves. Sunlight will not normally ignite the leaves, but if the same power is concentrated into a small area (increased intensity) by **focusing** with a magnifying glass, the leaves can be ignited. An effect is therefore produced by increasing the intensity even though the power remains the same.

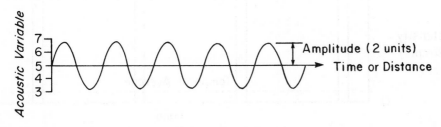

Figure 2.9. Amplitude is the maximum amount of variation that occurs in an acoustic variable. It is equal to the maximum value of the variable minus the normal value. In this figure, the amplitude is seven (maximum value) minus five (normal value); the amplitude is two units.

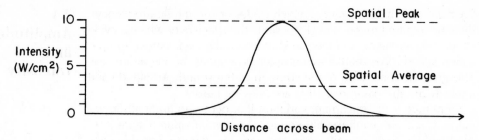

Figure 2.10. Intensity is a function of distance across beam. In this figure, spatial peak intensity (at the beam center) is 10 W/cm², spatial average is 3 W/cm², and the SP/SA factor is 3.3. In addition to varying across the beam, intensity varies along the direction of the beam.

We will see in Section 4.3 that beam area is determined in part by the size and **operating frequency** of the sound source chosen. For a given beam power, intensity will be determined by the beam area resulting from the choice of sound source.

Intensity is proportional to the square of amplitude. Thus if amplitude is doubled, intensity is quadrupled. If amplitude is halved, intensity is quartered.

Because intensity is not uniform across a sound beam (Figure 2.10) and, in the case of pulsed ultrasound, is not uniform in time (Figure 2.11), four intensities must be considered. For spatial considerations we may use either the spatial peak (SP) or spatial average (SA) value. These are related by the SP/SA factor.

$$\text{SP/SA factor} = \frac{\text{spatial peak intensity (W/cm}^2)}{\text{spatial average intensity (W/cm}^2)}$$

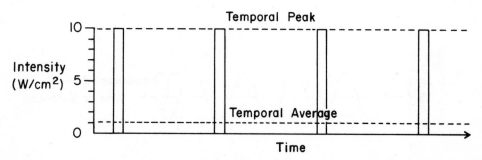

Figure 2.11. Intensity as a function of time for pulsed ultrasound. Temporal peak intensity (10 W/cm²) is the intensity when the sound is actually on. Temporal average intensity (1 W/cm²) is the intensity that results when this is averaged over time. In this figure, the duty factor is 0.1.

18

For temporal considerations, we may use either the temporal peak or temporal average value. These are related by the duty factor.

> temporal average intensity (W/cm) =
> duty factor × temporal peak intensity (W/cm²)

If the sound is continuous instead of pulsed, the duty factor is unity, and the temporal peak and temporal average intensities are equal to each other. The four intensities resulting from spatial and temporal considerations are spatial-average–temporal-average (SATA) intensity, spatial-peak–temporal-average (SPTA) intensity, spatial-average–temporal-peak (SATP) intensity, and spatial-peak–temporal-peak (SPTP) intensity. These are related to one another as shown in Table 2.1.

Usually, ultrasound pulses do not have constant amplitude and intensity within them, as shown in Figures 2.6 and 2.11. In this case the peak intensity occurring within each pulse is called the temporal peak intensity. The intensity averaged over the pulse duration is called the pulse average intensity (it is called temporal peak intensity elsewhere in this section, where pulses are assumed to have constant intensity within them).

Table 2.1
Process of Conversion from One Intensity to Another*

To convert	to	multiply (divide) by	and by
SATA	SPTA	SP/SA factor	1
	SATP	1	(duty factor)
	SPTP	SP/SA factor	(duty factor)
SPTA	SATA	(SP/SA factor)	1
	SATP	(SP/SA factor)	(duty factor)
	SPTP	1	(duty factor)
SATP	SATA	1	duty factor
	SPTA	SP/SA factor	duty factor
	SPTP	SP/SA factor	1
SPTP	SATA	(SP/SA factor)	duty factor
	SPTA	1	duty factor
	SATP	(SP/SA factor)	1

*For example, to convert SATA to SPTP, multiply by SP/SA factor and divide by duty factor. SATA: spatial-average–temporal-average intensity. SPTA: spatial-peak–temporal-average intensity. SATP: spatial-average–temporal-peak intensity. SPTP: spatial-peak–temporal-peak intensity.

Example
2.4.1

The SATA intensity is 1 mW/cm², the SP/SA factor is 10, and the duty factor is 0.002. Calculate SPTA, SATP, and SPTP intensities.

$$\text{SPTA intensity} = \text{SATA intensity} \times \text{SP/SA factor}$$
$$= 1 \times 10 = 10 \text{ mW/cm}^2$$

$$\text{SATP intensity} = \frac{\text{SATA intensity}}{\text{duty factor}}$$

$$= \frac{1}{0.002} = 500 \text{ mW/cm}^2$$

$$\text{SPTA intensity} = \frac{\text{SATA intensity} \times \text{SP/SA factor}}{\text{duty factor}}$$

$$= \frac{1 \times 10}{0.002} = 5000 \text{ mW/cm}^2 = 5 \text{ W/cm}^2$$

SATA intensity is the lowest of the four, and SPTP intensity is the highest. SPTA and SATP intensities have intermediate values with SATP normally being the greater of the two.

Exercises

2.4.1. Amplitude is the maximum _____ that occurs in an acoustic variable.

2.4.2. Intensity is the _____ in a wave divided by the beam _____.

2.4.3. The unit for intensity is _____.

2.4.4. Intensity is proportional to the square of

_____.

2.4.5. If power is doubled and beam area remains unchanged, intensity is _____.

2.4.6. If beam area is doubled and power remains unchanged, intensity is _____.

2.4.7. If both power and beam area are doubled, intensity is

_____.

2.4.8. If amplitude is doubled, intensity is

_____.

2.4.9. If a sound beam has a power of 10 mW and a beam area of 2 cm², the intensity is _____ mW/cm².

2.4.10. The SP/SA factor is the spatial _____ intensity divided by the spatial _____ intensity.

2.4.11. The duty factor is temporal _____ intensity divided by temporal _____ intensity.

2.4.12. Which of the following intensities are equal for continuous-wave sound?
a. spatial peak and average
b. temporal peak and average
c. spatial peak and temporal peak
d. spatial average and temporal average
e. none of the above

2.4.13. If the SATA intensity is 1 mW/cm², the SP/SA ratio is 3, and the duty factor is 0.001, calculate the following intensities:
a. SPTA: _____ mW/cm²
b. SATP: _____ W/cm²
C. SPTP: _____ W/cm²

2.4.14. If pulsed ultrasound is on 50 percent of the time (duty factor = 0.5) and temporal peak intensity is 4 mW/cm², temporal average intensity is _____ mW/cm².

2.4.15. If the maximum value of an acoustic variable is 10 units and the normal value is 7 units, the amplitude is _____ units.

The terms discussed previously (frequency, period, wavelength, propagation speed, amplitude, and intensity) describe sound waves. Two more terms are needed before we go on to a consideration of sound reflection (Chapter 3). They are **attenuation** and **impedance.** It is important to understand attenuation because it must be compensated for by the diagnostic instrument (Section 5.3).

For an unfocused beam (beams and focus are discussed in Chapter 4) in any real medium, like tissue, amplitude and intensity will decrease as the sound travels through the medium. This reduction in amplitude and intensity as sound travels is called attenuation (Figure 2.12). It encompasses **absorption** (conversion of sound to heat), reflection (Section 3.2), and **scattering** (Section 3.2). Attenuation units are **decibels (dB).** The **attenuation coefficient** is the attenuation per unit length of sound travel. Its units are decibels per centimeter (dB/cm). See Appendix 4 for a discussion of decibels. The longer the path over which the sound travels, the greater the attenuation.

2.5 Attenuation and Impedance

$$\text{attenuation (dB)} = \begin{array}{c}\text{attenuation coefficient (dB/cm)} \\ \times \text{ path length (cm)}\end{array}$$

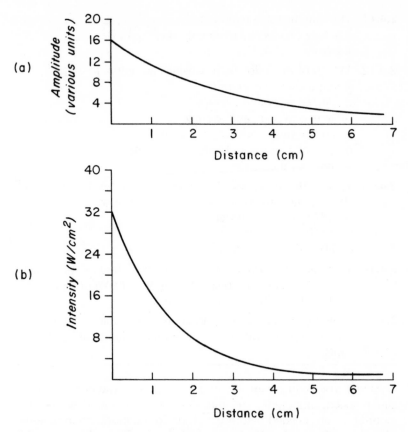

Figure 2.12. Attenuation of sound as it travels through a medium. Intensity decreases more rapidly than amplitude because it depends on the square of amplitude. In this figure, the amplitude decreases by 50 percent for each 2 cm of travel, and the intensity decreases by 50 percent for each 1 cm of travel. This corresponds to an attenuation coefficient of 3 dB/cm.

The attenuation coefficient increases with increasing frequency. Those who live in apartments or dormitories experience this fact by hearing mostly the bass notes through the wall from a neighbor's stereo system. For soft tissues, the attentuation coefficient depends on frequency in a linear fashion. A useful rule is that for average soft tissue there is 1 dB of attenuation per centimeter for each megahertz of frequency. The average attenuation coefficient in decibels per centimeter for soft tissues is equal to the frequency in MHz. In order to

> For soft tissues:
> attenuation coefficient (dB/cm) = frequency (MHz)

calculate the attenuation in decibels, simply multiply the frequency in megahertz (equal to attenuation coefficient in dB/cm) by the path length in centimeters, and the result is the attenuation in decibels.

> For soft tissues:
> attenuation (dB) = frequency (MHz) × path length (cm)

The intensity ratio corresponding to that number of decibels may be obtained from Table A4.1. This ratio is equal to the fraction of the intensity (at the beginning of the path) that remains at the end of the path. If the intensity at the beginning is known, the intensity at the end may be found by multiplying by the intensity ratio. This three-step process is repeated here:

1. Frequency (MHz) times path length (cm) yields attenuation (dB).
2. Find the intensity ratio in Table A4.1 for the decibel value calculated in Step 1.
3. The intensity ratio times the intensity at the start of the path equals the intensity at the end of the path.

Example 2.5.1

If 2-MHz ultrasound at 10 mW/cm² SATA intensity is applied to a soft-tissue surface, what is the SATA intensity 1.5 cm into the tissue? The frequency (MHz) multiplied by the path length (cm) is equal to 3. The attenuation is 3 dB. From Table A4.1 we find that 3 dB corresponds to an intensity ratio of 0.5. Thus, 50 percent of the intensity remains after the sound travels through this path. The intensity ratio (0.5) times the SATA intensity at the beginning of the path (10 mW/cm²) gives us the SATA intensity at the end of the path (5 mW/cm²).

Attenuation is higher in lung than in other soft tissues. In bone it is higher than in soft tissues. Lung and bone attenuations are not linearly dependent on frequency. Attenuation coefficient values for various tissues are given by Goss and associates.[5]

The depth of penetration is three times the reciprocal of the attenuation coefficient. It is given in centimeters and is defined as the depth at which intensity is reduced to 50 percent of its original value. It is therefore also the distance over which 50 percent of the original intensity is lost. This is also called the half-value layer or the half-value thickness. The depth of penetration decreases as frequency increases. It is useful

$$\text{depth of penetration (cm)} = \frac{3}{\text{attenuation coefficient (dB/cm)}}$$

For soft tissues:

$$\text{depth of penetration (cm)} = \frac{3}{\text{frequency (MHz)}}$$

when considering to what depths in tissue imaging may be accomplished.

We have discussed two characteristics of the medium through which sound travels: propagation speed and attenuation. A third characteristic, impedance, will be important for discussing reflections in the next chapter. Impedance is defined as the product of density and propagation speed. Its unit is the **rayl.** Impedance is determined by the density and stiffness of a medium. It increases if the density is increased or if the stiffness is increased.

> impedance (rayl) = density (kg/m³) × propagation speed (m/s)

Recall that propagation speed also depends on density and stiffness, but in a different way (Section 2.2).

Exercises

2.5.1. Attenuation is the reduction in _____ and _____ as a wave travels through a medium.

2.5.2. Attenuation consists of _____, _____, and _____.

2.5.3. The attenuation coefficient is attenuation per unit _____ of sound travel.

2.5.4. The attenuation and attenuation coefficient are given in the units _____ and _____, respectively.

2.5.5. For soft tissues, there is _____ dB of attenuation per centimeter for each megahertz of frequency.

2.5.6. For soft tissues the attenuation coefficient at 3 MHz is _____.

2.5.7. The attenuation coefficient in soft tissue _____ as frequency increases.

2.5.8. For soft tissue, if frequency is doubled, attenuation is _____; if path length is doubled, attenuation is _____; if both frequency and path length are doubled, attenuation is _____.

2.5.9. If frequency is doubled and path length is halved, attenuation is _____.

2.5.10. Absorption is the conversion of _____ to _____.

2.5.11. Can the absorption be greater than the attenuation in a given medium at a given frequency?

_____ .

2.5.12. Is attenuation in bone higher or lower than in soft tissue?

_____ .

2.5.13. For average soft tissue, the attenuation is such that for each 1.5 cm traveled, a 2-MHz sound intensity is reduced by _____ %; the depth of penetration is _____ cm. For 1 cm and 3 MHz, the reduction is _____ %, and the depth of penetration is _____ cm.

2.5.14. Impedance is the product of _____ and

_____ _____ .

2.5.15. If density and stiffness are increased, impedance is

_____ .

2.5.16. The attenuation coefficient for soft tissue at 5 MHz is _____ dB/cm.

2.5.17. The depth of penetration is three times the reciprocal of the

_____ _____ .

2.5.18. The depth of penetration _____ as frequency increases.

2.5.19. If the intensity of 2-MHz ultrasound entering soft tissue is 2 W/cm², the intensity at a depth of 4 cm is _____ W/cm². The depth of penetration is _____ cm.

2.5.20. If the intensity of 20-MHz ultrasound entering soft tissue is 2 W/cm², the intensity at a depth of 4 cm is

_____ W/cm.

2.5.21. If the density is 1000 kg/m³ and the propagation speed is 1.54 mm/µs, the impedance is _____ rayls.

Ultrasound is a wave of traveling acoustic variables: pressure, density, temperature, and particle motion. It is described by frequency, period, wavelength, propagation speed, amplitude, intensity, and attenuation. Pulsed ultrasound is described by additional terms: pulse repetition frequency, pulse repetition period, pulse duration, duty factor, and spatial pulse length. Propagation speed and impedance are characteristics of the medium that are determined by density and stiffness. Attenuation increases with frequency and path length. Depth of penetration decreases with increasing frequency. Four intensities (SATA, SPTA, SATP, and SPTP) are used to describe pulsed ultrasound. The soft-tissue propagation speed is 1.54 mm/µs, and the attenuation coefficient is 1 dB/cm for each megahertz of frequency.

2.6 Review

2.6.1. Which of the following is a characteristic of a medium through which sound is propagating?
a. impedance
b. intensity
c. amplitude
d. frequency
e. period

2.6.2. Which of the following applies to continuous-wave sound?
a. pulse duration
b. pulse repetition frequency
c. frequency
d. SP/SA factor
e. c and d

2.6.3. Match the following:
a. frequency: _____
b. period: _____
c. wavelength: _____
d. propagation speed: _____
e. amplitude: _____

1. time per cycle
2. maximum variation per cycle
3. length per cycle
4. cycles per second
5. speed of a wave through a medium

2.6.4. Match the following:
a. wavelength: _____
b. duty factor: _____
c. intensity: _____
d. SP/SA factor: _____

1. $\dfrac{\text{SPTA intensity}}{\text{SATA intensity}}$

2. $\dfrac{\text{propagation speed}}{\text{frequency}}$

3. $\dfrac{\text{pulse duration}}{\text{pulse repetition period}}$

4. $\dfrac{\text{power}}{\text{beam area}}$

2.6.5. Match the following:
a. period: _____
b. pulse repetition period: _____
c. impedance: _____
d. propagation speed: _____
e. depth of penetration: _____
f. pulse duration: _____
g. spatial pulse length: _____

1. density × propagation speed
2. frequency × wavelength
3. $\dfrac{1}{\text{frequency}}$
4. $\dfrac{1}{\text{pulse repetition frequency}}$
5. $\dfrac{3}{\text{attenuation coefficient}}$

6. number of cycles in the
   pulse × wavelength
7. number of cycles in the
   pulse × period

2.6.6. Match the following quantities with their units (answers may
be used more than once):

a. frequency: _____   1. s
b. wavelength: _____   2. mm/μs
c. period: _____   3. Hz
d. propagation speed: _____   4. mm
e. pulse duration: _____   5. W/cm²
f. pulse repetition frequency: 6. W
_____   7. dB/cm
g. pulse repetition period: 8. dB
_____   9. cm²
h. intensity: _____   10. cm
i. attenuation: _____
j. attenuation coefficient:

_____

k. power: _____
l. beam area: _____
m. depth of penetration: _____

2.6.7. Match the following (each answer should be used twice):

a. attenuation coefficient   1. soft tissues
   =1 dB/cm at 1 MHz: _____   2. lung
b. high attenuation: _____,   3. bone

_____

c. high propagation speed:

_____

d. propagation speed
   1.54 mm/μs: _____
e. low propagation speed:

_____

2.6.8. Given the following:

frequency = 2 MHz
pulse repetition frequency = 1 kHz
4 cycles per pulse
SATA intensity = 1 mW/cm²
SP/SA ratio = 4
density 1058 kg/m³
Applying these values to a soft-tissue surface, find the
following:
a. propagation speed: _____ mm/μs
b. wavelength: _____ mm

c. spatial pulse length: _____ mm
d. period: _____ μs
e. pulse duration: _____ μs
f. pulse repetition period: _____ ms
g. duty factor: _____
h. SPTP intensity at the surface: _____ W/cm²
i. attenuation coefficient: _____ dB/cm
j. depth of penetration: _____ cm
k. attenuation from surface to 3 cm depth: _____ dB
l. intensity ratio corresponding to dB in k:

_____

m. SATA intensity at 3 cm depth: _____
   mW/cm²
n. SPTA intensity at 3 cm depth: _____ mW/cm²
o. SATP intensity at 3 cm depth: _____
   mW/cm²
p. SPTP intensity at 3 cm depth: _____
   mW/cm²
q. impedance: _____ rayls

2.6.9. Which of the following is independent of the others?
a. frequency
b. period
c. amplitude
d. wavelength
e. propagation speed

2.6.10. Which of the following is independent of the others?
a. frequency
b. amplitude
c. intensity
d. power
e. beam area

Chapter 3

Reflection, Scattering, Refraction, and Doppler Effect

In Chapter 2 we considered the propagation of ultrasound through homogeneous media. The usefulness of ultrasound as an imaging tool is due primarily to reflection at organ boundaries and scattering within heterogeneous tissues. These phenomena will be considered in this chapter.

3.1 Introduction

Normal incidence occurs when the direction of travel of the ultrasound is perpendicular to the boundary between two media (Figure 3.1). If the incidence is not normal, it is called **oblique incidence.** This will be discussed in the next section.

When there is normal incidence, the incident sound may be reflected or transmitted or both (Figure 3.2). Reflected sound travels through medium one in a direction opposite to the incident sound (i.e., the reflected sound returns to the sound source). Transmitted sound moves through medium two in the same direction as the incident sound. The intensities of the reflected sound and transmitted sound depend on the incident intensity and the impedances (in rayls) of the media.

3.2 Normal Incidence and Scattering

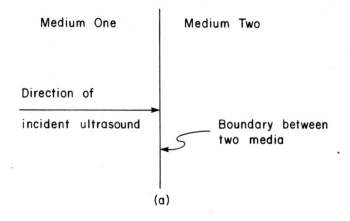

(a)

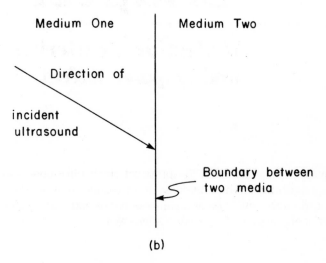

(b)

Figure 3.1. Normal incidence (a) and oblique incidence (b) at a boundary between two media.

With normal incidence:
  reflected intensity (W/cm²) = incident intensity (W/cm²) ×
  $\left[\dfrac{\text{medium two impedance} - \text{medium one impedance}}{\text{medium two impedance} + \text{medium one impedance}}\right]^{2}$
transmitted intensity (W/cm²) = incident intensity (W/cm²) −
                        reflected intensity (W/cm²)

We see that, for normal incidence, if the media impedances are the same, there is no reflected sound, and transmitted intensity is equal to incident intensity. If there is no reflection, we know that the media

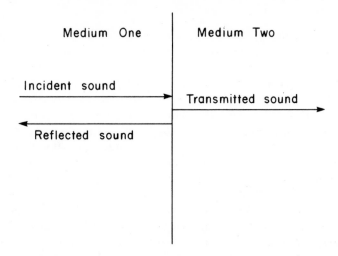

Figure 3.2. Reflection and transmission at a boundary with normal incidence. The lateral offset of transmitted and reflected sound with respect to incident sound is for figure clarity. An actual lateral shift does not occur.

impedances are equal. We see also that the reflected and transmitted intensities depend not only on the (subtraction) difference between the media impedances but also on their sum (compare Problems 3.2.4 and 3.2.5, where the impedance differences are the same, but the answers are different, and compare Problems 3.2.4 and 3.2.6, where impedance differences are different, but the answers are the same).

The reflected intensity divided by the incident intensity is called the **intensity reflection coefficient.** The transmitted intensity divided by the incident intensity is called the **intensity transmission coefficient.**

> With normal incidence:
> intensity reflection coefficient $= \dfrac{\text{reflected intensity (W/cm}^2)}{\text{incident intensity (W/cm}^2)}$
>
> $= \left[\dfrac{\text{medium two impedance } - \text{ medium one impedance}}{\text{medium two impedance } + \text{ medium one impedance}} \right]^2$
>
> intensity transmission coefficient $= \dfrac{\text{transmitted intensity (W/cm}^2)}{\text{incident intensity (W/cm}^2)}$
>
> $= 1 - \text{intensity reflection coefficient}$

Recall that impedance is the product of density and propagation speed. For normal incidence, a reflection is generated at a boundary if the impedances are different. A reflection may be generated when the densities are the same if the propagation speeds are different (see Problem 3.2.10). On the other hand, no reflection may be generated even when the densities are different (see Problem 3.2.11). If there is a large

31

difference between the impedances, there will be almost total reflection (intensity reflection coefficient close to unity). An example of this is an air/soft-tissue boundary (see Problem 3.2.17). For this reason, a **coupling medium** (an oil or a gel) is used to provide a good sound path from the source to the skin during the diagnostic use of ultrasound.

In the preceding discussion and in the following section it is assumed that wavelength is small compared with the boundary dimensions. The resulting reflections are called **specular reflections.** If, on the other hand, the boundary dimensions are comparable to or small compared with the wavelength, or if the boundary is not smooth, the incident sound will be scattered (diffused). Scattering is the redirection of sound in many directions by rough surfaces or by heterogeneous media such as (cellular) tissues or particle suspensions such as blood. **Backscatter** (sound scattered back in the direction from which it originally came) intensities from rough surfaces and heterogeneous media vary with frequency and scatterer size. They may be comparable to or less than specular reflection intensities from tissue boundaries. The roughness of a tissue boundary effectively increases as frequency is increased (increased backscatter). This helps to make echo reception less dependent on **incidence angle** (see Figures 3.3 and 4.10).

Exercises

3.2.1. When ultrasound encounters a boundary with normal incidence, the _____ of the tissues must be different to produce a reflection.

3.2.2. With normal incidence, two media _____ and the incident _____ must be known in order to calculate reflected intensity.

3.2.3. With normal incidence, two media _____ must be known in order to calculate the intensity reflection coefficient.

3.2.4. For an incident intensity of 2 mW/cm² and impedances of 49 and 51 rayls, the reflected intensity is _____ mW/cm², and the transmitted intensity is _____ mW/cm².

3.2.5. For an incident intensity of 2 mW/cm² and impedances of 99 and 101 rayls, the reflected and transmitted intensities are _____ and _____ mW/cm².

3.2.6. For an incident intensity of 2 mW/cm² and impedances of 98 and 102 rayls, the reflected and transmitted intensities are _____ and _____ mW/cm².

3.2.7. For an incident intensity of 5 mW/cm² and impedances of 45 and 55 rayls, the intensity reflection coefficient is _____ .

3.2.8. For impedances of 45 and 55 rayls, the intensity transmission coefficient is _____ .

3.2.9. For impedances of 45 and 55 rayls, the intensity reflection coefficient is _____ dB.

3.2.10. Given the following:
incident intensity = 1 mW/cm²
medium one:
   density = 1.0 kg/m³
   propagation speed = 1350 m/s
medium two:
   density = 1.0 kg/m³
   propagation speed = 1650 m/s
The reflected intensity is _____ mW/cm².

3.2.11. Given the following:
incident intensity = 5 mW/cm²
medium one:
   density = 1.00 kg/m³
   propagation speed = 1515 m/s
medium two:
   density = 1.01 kg/m³
   propagation speed = 1500 m/s
The reflected intensity is _____ mW/cm².

3.2.12. Given the following:
incident intensity = 5 mW/cm²
medium one impedance = 2 rayls
medium two impedance = 0 rayls
The reflected and transmitted intensities are _____ and _____ mW/cm².

3.2.13. If the media impedances are equal, there is no reflection. True or false?

3.2.14. If the media densities are equal, there is no reflection. True or false?

3.2.15. Redirection of sound in many directions as it encounters rough media junctions or particle suspensions is called _____ .

3.2.16. The intensity reflection and transmission coefficients depend on whether the sound is traveling from medium one into medium two or vice versa. True or false?

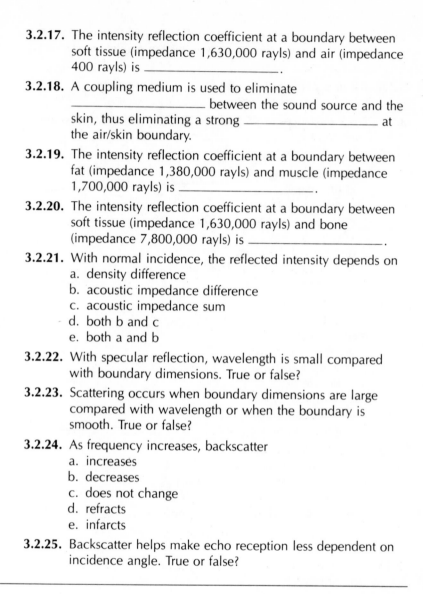

3.2.17. The intensity reflection coefficient at a boundary between soft tissue (impedance 1,630,000 rayls) and air (impedance 400 rayls) is _____.

3.2.18. A coupling medium is used to eliminate _____ between the sound source and the skin, thus eliminating a strong _____ at the air/skin boundary.

3.2.19. The intensity reflection coefficient at a boundary between fat (impedance 1,380,000 rayls) and muscle (impedance 1,700,000 rayls) is _____.

3.2.20. The intensity reflection coefficient at a boundary between soft tissue (impedance 1,630,000 rayls) and bone (impedance 7,800,000 rayls) is _____.

3.2.21. With normal incidence, the reflected intensity depends on
a. density difference
b. acoustic impedance difference
c. acoustic impedance sum
d. both b and c
e. both a and b

3.2.22. With specular reflection, wavelength is small compared with boundary dimensions. True or false?

3.2.23. Scattering occurs when boundary dimensions are large compared with wavelength or when the boundary is smooth. True or false?

3.2.24. As frequency increases, backscatter
a. increases
b. decreases
c. does not change
d. refracts
e. infarcts

3.2.25. Backscatter helps make echo reception less dependent on incidence angle. True or false?

3.3
Oblique
Incidence
and
Refraction

Oblique incidence occurs when the direction of travel of the ultrasound is not perpendicular to the boundary between two media (Figure 3.1). The direction of travel with respect to the boundary is given by the incidence angle (for normal incidence, the incidence angle is zero, Section 3.2). The reflected and transmitted directions are given by the **reflection angle** and **transmission angle,** respectively (Figure 3.3). They are related as follows:

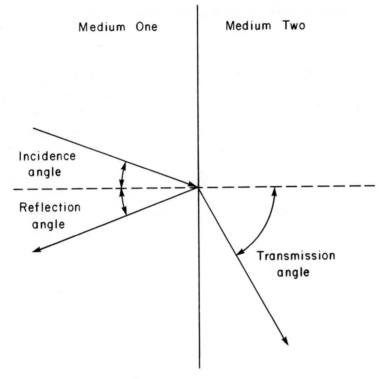

Figure 3.3. Reflection and transmission at a boundary with oblique incidence. Incidence and reflection angles are equal. The transmission angle depends on the incidence angle and the media propagation speeds.

reflection angle (°) = incidence angle (°)

sine of transmission angle (°) = sine of incidence angle (°) ×

$$\left[\frac{\text{medium two propagation speed (mm/}\mu\text{s)}}{\text{medium one propagation speed (mm/}\mu\text{s)}} \right]$$

The second equation is called **Snell's law.** See Appendix 3 for a discussion of the **sine** of an angle. A change in direction of sound when crossing a boundary is called **refraction.** The transmission angle is greater than the incidence angle if the propagation speed through medium two is greater than the propagation speed through medium one [Figure 3.4(a)]. There is no refraction if the propagation speeds are equal [Figure 3.4(b)] or if the incidence angle is zero (normal incidence).

Expressions for calculating reflected and transmitted intensities are more complicated than those that apply when there is normal incidence, and they are not given here. For given media, the reflection

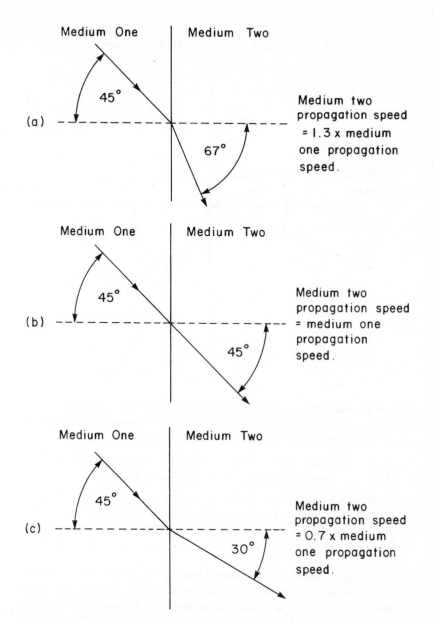

Figure 3.4. Transmission angles for an incidence angle of 45 degrees and propagation speeds through medium two greater than (a), equal to (b), and less than (c) propagation speeds through medium one.

coefficient for oblique incidence may be smaller than, equal to, or greater than that for normal incidence, depending on incidence angle. If the propagation speeds through the media are the same, the intensity reflection coefficient is the same as that for normal incidence (see Section 3.2) and is independent of incidence angle. For oblique incidence it is possible for a reflection to occur even if the media have equal impedances. This will occur if the propagation speeds are different. Conversely, it is possible that no reflection will occur even when the media impedances are different. Therefore, absence of reflection with oblique incidence does not necessarily mean that the media impedances are equal (as it did with normal incidence).

Exercises

3.3.1. Refraction is a change in _____ of sound when it crosses a boundary.

3.3.2. If the propagation speed through medium two is larger than the propagation speed through medium one, the transmission angle will be _____ _____ the incidence angle, and the reflection angle will be _____ _____ the incidence angle.

3.3.3. If the propagation speed through medium two is smaller than the propagation speed through medium one, the transmission angle will be _____ _____ the incidence angle, and the reflection angle will be _____ _____ the incidence angle.

3.3.4. If the propagation speed through medium two is equal to the propagation speed through medium one, the transmission angle will be _____ _____ the incidence angle, and the reflection angle will be _____ _____ the incidence angle.

3.3.5. If the incidence angle is 30 degrees, the propagation speed through medium one is 1000 m/s, and the propagation speed through medium two is 700 m/s, the reflection angle is _____ degrees, and the transmission angle is _____ degrees.

3.3.6. If the incidence angle is 30 degrees, the propagation speed through medium one is 1000 m/s, and the propagation speed through medium two is 1000 m/s, the reflection angle is _____ degrees, and the transmission angle is _____ degrees.

3.3.7. If the incidence angle is 30 degrees and the propagation speed through medium two is 30 percent higher than the propagation speed through medium one, the reflection angle is _____ degrees, and the transmission angle is _____ degrees.

3.3.8. Given the following:
   incidence angle = 20 degrees
   incident intensity = 5 mW/cm²
   propagation speed through medium one = 1500 m/s
   impedance of medium one = 8 rayls
   propagation speed through medium two = 1500 m/s
   impedance of medium two = 12 rayls
   The reflection coefficient is _____.

3.3.9. Given the following:
   incidence angle = 20 degrees
   incident intensity = 5 mW/cm²
   transmission angle = 20 degrees
   impedance of medium one = 8 rayls
   impedance of medium two = 12 rayls
   The reflected intensity is _____
   mW/cm².

3.3.10. Under what two conditions does refraction not occur?
   a. _____
   b. _____

3.3.11. Under what condition is the reflection coefficient not dependent on incidence angle?

   _____

3.3.12. When ultrasound encounters a boundary at an oblique incidence, either _____ or
   _____ _____ must
   change in order to generate a reflection.

3.3.13. The low speed of sound in fat is a major source of image degradation due to refraction. If the incidence angle at a boundary between fat (1450 m/s) and kidney (1561 m/s) is 30 degrees, the transmission angle is _____ degrees.

3.4 Doppler Effect

Thus far in this chapter we have considered only media boundaries that are stationary with respect to the sound source. If a boundary is moving with respect to the source, the **Doppler effect** will occur. The Doppler effect is a change in reflected frequency caused by **reflector** motion. If the media boundary (reflector) is moving toward the source [Figure 3.5(a)], the reflected frequency will be higher than the incident frequency. If the reflector is moving away from the source [Figure 3.5(b)], the reflected frequency will be lower than the incident frequency. The greater the speed of the boundary, the greater will be the difference between incident and reflected frequencies.

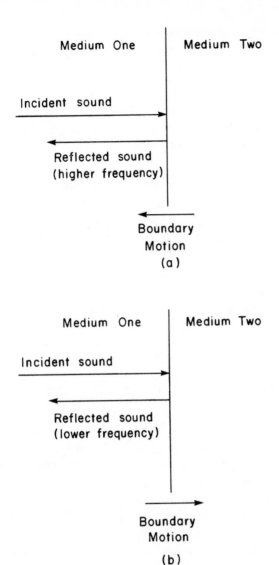

Figure 3.5. Doppler effect. (a) If the reflector (boundary) moves toward the source, the reflected frequency is higher than the incident frequency. (b) If the reflector moves away from the source, the reflected frequency is lower than the incident frequency.

reflected frequency (MHz) = incident frequency (MHz) $\times$

$$\left[1 \pm \frac{2 \times \text{reflector speed (m/s)}}{\text{propagation speed (m/s)} + \text{reflector speed (m/s)}} \right]$$

The plus sign is used when the reflector is moving toward the source, and the minus sign is used when the reflector is moving away from the source. If the direction of the incident sound is not parallel to the boundary motion, the last term in parentheses on the right-hand side of the preceding equation must be multiplied by the **cosine** of the angle between these directions. See Appendix 3 for a discussion of the cosine of an angle. The incident frequency subtracted from the reflected frequency is called the **Doppler shift.**

Doppler shift (MHz) = reflected frequency (MHz) − incident frequency (MHz) =

$$\pm \ \frac{2 \times \text{reflector speed (m/s)} \times \text{incident frequency (MHz)}}{\text{propagation speed (m/s)} + \text{reflector speed (m/s)}}$$

An instrument designed to measure the difference between the incident and reflected frequencies can yield information on reflector motion. The moving reflector could be a tissue boundary (e.g., a blood vessel wall or fetal heart) or a cell in suspension (e.g., blood cells in circulation).

Exercises

3.4.1. The Doppler effect is a change in reflected _____ caused by reflector _____ .

3.4.2. If the reflector is moving toward the source, the reflected frequency is _____ than the incident frequency.

3.4.3. If the reflector is moving away from the source, the reflected frequency is _____ than the incident frequency.

3.4.4. If the reflector is stationary with respect to the source, the reflected frequency is _____ _____ the incident frequency.

3.4.5. Measurement of Doppler shift yields information about reflector _____ .

3.4.6. If the incident frequency is 1 MHz, the propagation speed is 1600 m/s, and the reflector speed is 16 m/s toward the source, the reflected frequency is _____ MHz.

3.4.7. If 2-MHz ultrasound is reflected from a soft-tissue boundary moving at 10 m/s toward the source, the Doppler shift is _____ MHz.

3.4.8. If 2-MHz ultrasound is reflected from a soft-tissue boundary moving at 10 m/s away from the source, the Doppler shift is _____ MHz.

3.4.9. Doppler shift is the difference between _____ and _____ frequencies.

3.4.10. When incident sound direction and reflector motion are not parallel, calculation of the reflected frequency involves the _____ of the angle between these directions.

3.4.11. If the angle between incident sound direction and reflector motion is 60 degrees, the reflected frequency in Problem 3.4.6 is _____ MHz.

In Section 2.5, attenuation (reduction in intensity as sound travels) was discussed. We saw that for soft tissues there is 1 dB of attenuation per centimeter for each 1 MHz of frequency. In Sections 3.2 and 3.3, reflection at media boundaries was discussed. In Problem 3.2.9, the reflection coefficient was calculated in decibels. We shall now consider the situation in which these effects are combined. To calculate the intensity of reflections received at the surface (Figure 3.6), attenuation and the reflection coefficient must both be taken into account. The procedure used is illustrated in the following examples.

3.5 Attenuation and Reflection Combined

If 10-mW/cm² ultrasound applied to the surface of a medium with an attenuation coefficient of 2.5 dB/cm travels to a boundary at a depth of 2 cm where the impedances are 0.75 and 0.25 rayls, and the reflected sound travels 2 cm back to the surface, what is the intensity of the sound received at the surface? To solve this problem, we calculate the attenuation (dB) occurring on the 2-cm trip to the reflector, the reflection coefficient (dB), and the attenuation (dB) occurring on the 2-cm return trip to the surface. The attenuation (dB) is the same for both trips. We multiply the attenuation coefficient (dB/cm) by the path length (cm) to get the attenuation (dB). For each trip this is 2.5 dB/cm times 2 cm, which is 5 dB. The reflection coefficient is

Example 3.5.1

$$\left[\frac{0.25 - 0.75}{0.25 + 0.75} \right]^2 = 0.25$$

The transmission coefficient is 0.75, but that is not needed in this example. The reflection coefficient (Table A4.1) is 6 dB. The sum of 5 dB (attenuation for trip to the reflector), 6 dB (reflection), and 5 dB (attenu-

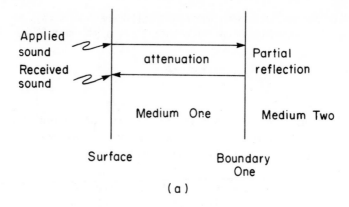

(a)

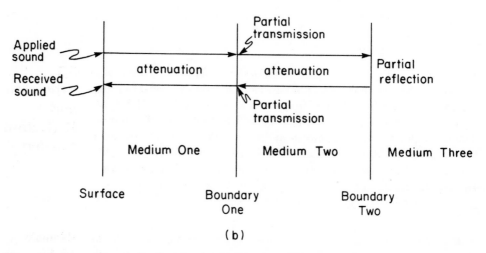

(b)

Figure 3.6. Attenuation and reflection combined. (a) Reflection at boundary one. The applied sound travels through medium one, with attenuation, to boundary one, where the first reflection is produced. The reflection returns to the surface through medium one, with attenuation. For this case, reduction in received intensity is caused by (1) attenuation on the trip to boundary one, (2) partial (incomplete) reflection at boundary one, and (3) attenuation on the return trip to the surface. (b) Reflection at boundary two. The applied sound travels through medium one, with attenuation, to boundary one, where partial transmission (and the first reflection) occur. The sound transmitted into medium two travels, with attenuation, to boundary two, where the second (partial) reflection is generated. It returns to boundary one through medium two, with attenuation. At boundary one, the second reflection is partially transmitted. The portion transmitted into medium one travels, with attenuation, back to the surface. For this case, reduction in received intensity is caused by (1) attenuation on the trip to boundary one, (2) partial transmission at boundary one, (3) attenuation on the trip to boundary two, (4) partial reflection at boundary two, (5) attenuation on the return trip to boundary one, (6) partial transmission at boundary one, and (7) attenuation on the return trip to the surface.

ation for trip to the surface) is 16 dB. This corresponds to an intensity ratio of 0.025. The intensity received at the surface is then

$$10 \text{ mW/cm}^2 \text{ (applied intensity)} \times 0.025 \text{ (intensity ratio)} = 0.25 \text{ mW/cm}^2$$

If 10-mW/cm² ultrasound is applied to a surface, travels through a medium with an impedance of 0.75 rayls and an attenuation coefficient of 2.5 dB/cm to a boundary at a depth of 1 cm, then travels 1 cm through a medium with an impedance of 0.25 rayls and an attenuation coefficient of 2.5 dB/cm to a second boundary where the third impedance is 0.75 rayls, what is the intensity at the surface resulting from the reflection at the second boundary? The total attenuation due to travel to the second boundary and back is 2.5 dB/cm $\times$ 4 cm, or 10 dB. The reflection coefficient at the first boundary is

Example 3.5.2

$$\left[\frac{0.25 - 0.75}{0.25 + 0.75} \right]^2 = 0.25$$

The transmission coefficient is 0.75. From Table A4.1 this is found to be approximately 1 dB (intensity ratio 0.79). The reflection coefficient at the second boundary is

$$\left[\frac{0.75 - 0.25}{0.75 + 0.25} \right]^2 = 0.25 \text{ (6 dB)}$$

The reflection coefficient at the first boundary (encountered by the reflected sound from the second boundary on its return trip to the surface) is

$$\left[\frac{0.75 - 0.25}{0.75 + 0.25} \right]^2 = 0.25$$

Again the transmission coefficient is 0.75 (1 dB). Here the role of the impedances is reversed, since the reflected sound (from the second boundary) is traveling from the second medium into the first. However, the reflection and transmission coefficients are the same as calculated before. The combined decibels of attenuation and reflection are:

$$10 \text{ dB (round-trip attenuation)} +$$
$$2 \text{ dB (two transmissions at boundary one)} +$$
$$6 \text{ dB (one reflection at boundary two)} = 18 \text{ dB}$$

This corresponds to an intensity ratio of 0.016. Thus the received intensity at the surface from a reflection at the second boundary is

$$10 \text{ mW/cm}^2 \times 0.016 = 0.16 \text{ mW/cm}^2$$

Example 3.5.3   If 10-mW/cm² 2.5-MHz ultrasound is applied to a soft-tissue surface, travels through a soft-tissue impedance of 1,440,000 rayls to a boundary at a depth of 1 cm, then travels 1 cm through a soft-tissue impedance of 1,760,000 rayls to a second boundary where the third impedance is 1,440,000 rayls, what is the intensity at the surface resulting from the reflection at the second boundary? Since soft tissues are involved (Section 2.5), the total attenuation due to travel to the second boundary and back is 2.5 MHz × 4 cm, or 10 dB. The reflection coefficient at the first boundary is

$$\left[\frac{1,760,000 - 1,440,000}{1,760,000 + 1,440,000}\right]^2 = 0.01$$

The transmission coefficient is 0.99 (0 dB). The reflection coefficient at the second boundary is

$$\left[\frac{1,440,000 - 1,760,000}{1,440,000 + 1,760,000}\right]^2 = 0.01 \ (20 \ dB)$$

The reflection coefficient at the first boundary (encountered by the reflected sound from the second boundary on its return trip to the surface) is

$$\left[\frac{1,440,000 - 1,760,000}{1,440,000 + 1,760,000}\right]^2 = 0.01$$

Again the transmission coefficient is 0.99 (0 dB). Here the role of the impedances is reversed, since the reflected sound (from the second boundary) is traveling from the second medium into the first. However, the reflection and transmission coefficients are the same as calculated before. The combined decibels of attenuation and reflection are

10 dB (round-trip attenuation) + 0 dB (two transmissions) + 20 dB (one reflection) = 30 dB

This corresponds to an intensity ratio of 0.001. Thus the received intensity at the surface from a reflection at the second boundary is

10 mW/cm² × 0.001 = 0.01 mW/cm²

Exercises

3.5.1. For 5-MHz sound passing through 2 cm of soft tissue to a boundary where impedances are 1,350,000 and 1,650,000 rayls and returning to the surface, the combined decibels of attenuation and reflection are _____ dB.

3.5.2. If the applied intensity in Problem 3.5.1 is 1mW/cm², the received intensity at the surface is _____ mW/cm².

3.5.3. For 5-MHz sound (applied intensity 1 mW/cm²) traveling 2 cm through soft tissue to a boundary where impedances are 1,350,000 and 1,650,000 rayls and then 1 cm to a second boundary where impedances are 1,650,000 and 550,000 rayls, the received intensities for both reflections are _____ and _____ mW/cm².

3.5.4. For sound of initial intensity 1 mW/cm² traveling 2 cm through tissue with an attenuation coefficient of 3 dB/cm to a boundary where impedances are 1,350,000 and 1,650,000 rayls and then 1 cm through tissue with an attenuation coefficient of 7 dB/cm to a second boundary where impedances are 1,650,000 and 550,000 rayls, the received intensities (at the starting point) for both reflections are _____ and _____ mW/cm².

3.6 Range Equation and Multiple Reflections

Now that we have considered sound propagation and reflection, we can learn about a very important consideration for **pulse-echo diagnostic ultrasound:** the **range equation.** The approach in pulse-echo diagnostic ultrasound is (1) to generate short pulses of sound that travel through the body, producing reflections **(echoes)** that travel back to the source and (2) to detect and display the returning echoes. The method that the instrumentation uses to properly position the echo on the display will be described in Section 5.4. The two items of information required are (1) the direction from which the echo came (assumed to be the direction in which the source is pointed) and (2) the distance to the boundary (reflecting surface or reflector) where the echo was produced. The distance is calculated from the range (distance-to-reflector) equation:

$$\text{distance to reflector (mm)} = \tfrac{1}{2}\,[\text{propagation speed (mm/}\mu s) \times \text{pulse round-trip time (}\mu s)]$$

To get the distance from the source to the reflector, the propagation speed in the intervening medium must be known or assumed, and the pulse round-trip time must be measured. The reason that the factor ½ appears is that the round-trip time is the time for the pulse to travel to the reflector and return; we desire only the distance to the reflector. The soft-tissue average propagation speed (1.54 mm/μs) is usually as-

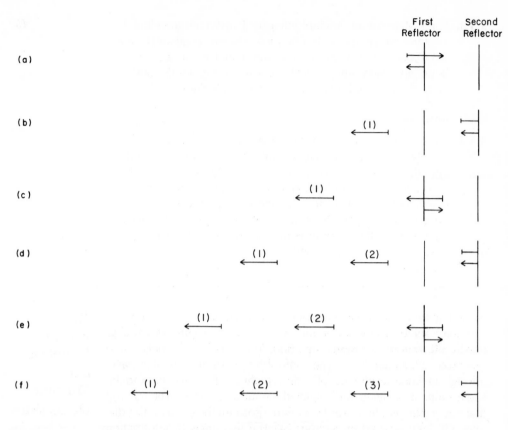

Figure 3.7. The generation of multiple reflections (reverberations). (a) An ultrasound pulse has come from the left, has encountered the first reflector, and has been partially reflected and partially transmitted. (b) Reflection and transmission at the first reflector are complete. Reflection at the second reflector is occurring. (c) Reflection at the second reflector is complete. Partial transmission (from right to left this time) and partial reflection are again occurring at the first reflector. (d) The reflections from the first (1) and second (2) reflectors are traveling to the left toward the sound source. A second reflection [repeat of (b)] is occurring at the second reflector. (e) Partial transmission and reflection are again occurring at the first reflector. (f) Three reflections are now traveling to the left: (1) is the reflection from the first reflector; (2) is the reflection from the second reflector; (3) is the reflection from the second reflector, reflected from the back side of the first reflector (c) and reflected again from the second reflector (d). A fourth reflection is being generated at the second reflector.

sumed in using the range equation (unless another speed is given). For this case:

> For soft tissues:
> distance to reflector (mm) = 0.77 × pulse round-trip time (μs)

If two or more reflectors are encountered in the sound path, **multiple reflections (reverberations)** will occur. These may be sufficiently

strong to be detected by the instrumentation and to cause confusion on
the display. The process by which they are produced is shown in Figure 3.7. Multiple reflections will be discussed further in Section 5.7.

Exercises

3.6.1. The approach in pulse-echo ultrasound is (1) to generate
_____ of sound that travel through the body,
producing _____ that travel back to the
source, and (2) to detect and _____ the
returning echoes.

3.6.2. To calculate the distance to a reflector, we must know the
_____ _____ and the pulse
round-trip _____ .

3.6.3. If the propagation speed is 1.6 mm/μs and the pulse
round-trip time is 5 μs, the distance to the reflector is _____
mm.

3.6.4. If the propagation speed is 1.4 mm/μs and the time for a
pulse to travel to the reflector is 5 μs, the distance to the
reflector is _____ mm.

3.6.5. When the pulse round-trip time is 10 μs, the distance to a
reflector in soft tissue is _____ mm.

3.6.6. When the pulse round-trip time is 13 μs, the distance to a
reflector in soft tissue is _____ cm.

3.6.7. Multiple reflections are also called _____ .

3.6.8. Reverberation causes us to think there are reflectors that are
too great in
    a. impedance
    b. attenuation
    c. amplitude
    d. size
    e. number

3.6.9. Reverberation results when _____ or more
reflectors are in the sound path.

If two reflectors are encountered along the sound path, but they are not
sufficiently separated, they will not produce separate reflections and
thus will not be separated on the instrumentation display. The important parameter in determining the required separation is the spatial
pulse length (Section 2.3). The **longitudinal** resolution is the minimum
reflector separation required along the direction of sound travel so that
separate reflections will be produced (Figure 3.8). It is also called axial,
range, or depth resolution:

**3.7
Longitudinal
Resolution
and
Useful
Frequency
Range**

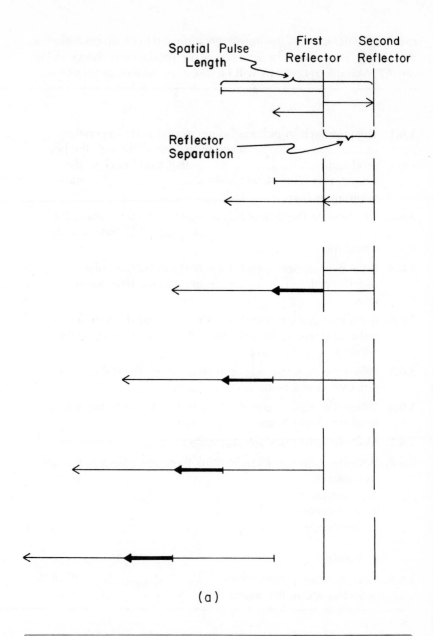

Spatial Pulse Length

First Reflector

Second Reflector

Reflector Separation

(a)

longitudinal resolution (mm) = $\dfrac{\text{spatial pulse length (mm)}}{2}$

For soft tissues:

longitudinal resolution (mm) = $\dfrac{0.77 \times \text{number of cycles in the pulse}}{\text{frequency (MHz)}}$

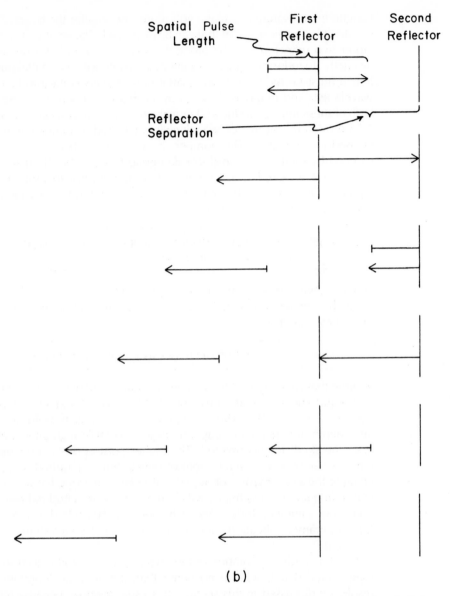

Spatial Pulse Length

First Reflector

Second Reflector

Reflector Separation

(b)

Figure 3.8. Longitudinal resolution. (a) The separation of the reflectors is less than half the spatial pulse length, so that reflection overlap occurs. Separate reflections are not produced. The reflectors are not resolved. (b) The separation of the reflectors is greater than half the spatial pulse length, so that reflection overlap does not occur. Separate reflections are produced, and the reflectors are resolved. Action proceeds in time from top to bottom in each part of the figure.

Longitudinal resolution is like a golf score: the smaller the better. The smaller it is, the more detail that can be displayed. The smaller it is, the closer two reflectors can be along the sound path and still be seen distinctly. To reduce (improve) longitudinal resolution, the spatial pulse length must be reduced. Since spatial pulse length is the product of wavelength and number of cycles in the pulse (Section 2.3), one or both of these must be reduced. For a given propagation speed (such as 1.54 mm/μs in soft tissue), wavelength is reduced as frequency is increased (Section 2.2). The number of cycles in each pulse may be reduced by increasing transducer **damping;** this will be discussed in Section 4.2. If we reduce the number of cycles per pulse to a minimum (approximately three), the only way to further improve longitudinal resolution is to increase frequency:

> Longitudinal resolution decreases (improves) as frequency increases.

However, when this is done, there is a price to be paid. It is a reduction in depth of penetration (Section 2.5), because attenuation increases as frequency increases:

> Depth of penetration decreases as frequency increases.

In order that we may reasonably meet resolution and depth-of-penetration requirements, we are thus restricted to a useful frequency range between 1 and 10 MHz. The lower portion of the range is useful where large depth of penetration (e.g., an obese subject) or high attenuation (e.g., the skull) is encountered. The higher portion of the frequency range is useful where small depth of penetration is required (e.g., in imaging the eye, thyroid, or superficial vessels or in pediatric imaging). If frequencies less than 1 MHz are used, the longitudinal resolution is not sufficient. If frequencies higher than 10 MHz (less than 10 MHz in many applications) are used, the depth of penetration is not sufficient.

The longitudinal resolution of the imaging system (ability to display longitudinal detail) will be no better than the acoustic longitudinal resolution discussed in this section. It is usually worse, because electronics and the display can degrade resolution.

Exercises

3.7.1. Longitudinal resolution is the minimum reflector separation required along the direction of _____ _____ so that separate _____ are produced.

3.7.2. Longitudinal resolution depends directly on
_____ _____
_____ .

3.7.3. The smaller the longitudinal resolution is, the better it is. True or false?

3.7.4. If there are three cycles of wavelength 1 mm in a pulse, the longitudinal resolution is _____ mm.

3.7.5. For pulses traveling through soft tissue where frequency is 3 MHz and there are 4 cycles per pulse, the longitudinal resolution is _____ mm.

3.7.6. If there are three cycles per pulse, the longitudinal resolution in soft tissue at the extremes of the useful frequency range for diagnostic ultrasound are _____ and _____ mm.

3.7.7. Doubling the frequency causes longitudinal resolution to be
_____ .

3.7.8. Doubling the number of cycles per pulse causes longitudinal resolution to be _____ .

3.7.9. When studying an obese subject, a higher frequency will likely be required. True or false?

3.7.10. If better resolution is desired, a lower frequency will help. True or false?

3.7.11. If frequencies less than _____ MHz are used, longitudinal resolution is not sufficient.

3.7.12. If frequencies higher than _____ MHz are used, depth of penetration is not sufficient.

3.7.13. Increasing the frequency improves resolution because
_____ is reduced, thus reducing
_____ _____
_____ .

3.7.14. Increasing the frequency decreases the depth of penetration because _____ is increased.

When sound encounters (with _normal incidence_) boundaries between media whose impedances are different, part of the sound is reflected and part is transmitted. If the two media have the same impedance, there is no reflection. With _oblique incidence,_ the sound is refracted at a boundary between media where propagation speeds are different. Incidence and reflection angles are always equal. There may be a re-

**3.8
Review**

flection when the impedances are equal (if the propagation speeds are different), and there may not be a reflection even if the impedances are different. If a boundary is moving with respect to the source, the incident and reflected frequencies will differ. To calculate the intensity of received reflections, both attenuation and reflection coefficient must be taken into account. The range equation is used to determine distance to reflectors. Reverberations are generated between reflectors. Longitudinal resolution depends on spatial pulse length. The useful diagnostic ultrasound frequency range is 1 to 10 MHz.

Exercises

3.8.1. A two-cycle pulse of 5-MHz ultrasound produces separate reflections from reflectors in soft tissue separated by 1 mm. True or false?

3.8.2. The lower and upper limits of the frequency range useful in diagnostic ultrasound are determined by _____ and _____ _____ _____ requirements, respectively.

3.8.3. The range of frequencies useful for diagnostic ultrasound is _____ to _____ MHz.

3.8.4. If no refraction occurs as an oblique sound beam passes through the boundary between two materials, the _____ _____ of the materials are known to be _____.

3.8.5. What must be known in order to calculate distance to a reflector?
a. attenuation, speed, density
b. attenuation, impedance
c. attenuation, absorption
d. travel time, speed
e. density, speed

3.8.6. With normal incidence, if the impedances of two media are the same, there will be no
a. inflation
b. reflection
c. refraction
d. calibration
e. both b and c

3.8.7. What is the transmitted intensity if the incident intensity is 1 and the impedances are 1.00 and 2.64?
a. 0.2
b. 0.4
c. 0.6
d. 0.8
e. 1.0

3.8.8. If the incident intensity is 1 and the impedances are 3 and 2, the reflected intensity is _____.

3.8.9. If pulses of three cycles of 5-MHz ultrasound travel through 4 cm of soft tissue to a boundary with impedances of 4.5 and 5.5, _____ percent of the original sound intensity will be found in the returning echoes at the starting point.

3.8.10. For pulses returning from a boundary at 3 cm from the source, where impedances are 4.5 and 5.5 rayls, and
spatial pulse length = 3 mm
cycles per pulse = 2
propagation speed = 1.5 mm/μs
intensity at the source = 4 mW/cm^2
The intensity is _____ mW/cm^2. Assume soft-tissue attenuation.

3.8.11. No reflection will occur with normal incidence if the media _____ are equal.

3.8.12. No reflection will occur with oblique incidence if the media _____ are equal and the media _____ _____ are equal.

Chapter 4

Transducers and Sound Beams

4.1 Introduction

The characteristics of ultrasound that are important for diagnosis have been described in Chapters 2 and 3. In this chapter we shall describe the devices that generate and receive ultrasound. They form the connecting link (Figure 1.2) between the ultrasound/tissue interactions of Figure 1.1 and the instrumentation described in Chapter 5. Except for reference to sound beams in Section 2.4, we have not yet considered the confining of sound to beams. The devices described in this chapter do not produce sound that travels uniformly in all directions away from the source; rather, this sound is confined in beams, which will be described in Section 4.3.

4.2 Transducers

Transducers convert one form of energy (Section A2.6) to another. Examples are given in Table 4.1. **Ultrasound transducers** have no special name applied to them such as microphone or loudspeaker, the names applied to devices that accomplish similar functions with audible sound. Ultrasound transducers convert electrical energy into ultrasound energy and vice versa. Electrical voltages applied to them are converted to ultrasound. Ultrasound incident on them produces electrical voltages.

Ultrasound transducers operate on the **piezoelectricity** (from Greek: pressure-electricity) principle, which was discovered in the latter part of the nineteenth century. The principle is that some materials

Table 4.1
Transducer Examples

Transducer	converts	to
Light bulb	electricity	light and heat
Automobile engine	chemical energy	motion and heat
Ear	sound	nerve impulses
Oven	electricity	heat
Motor	electricity	motion
Generator	motion	electricity
Battery	chemical energy	electricity
Human	chemical energy	heat and motion
Microphone	audible sound	electricity
Loudspeaker	electricity	audible sound

(ceramics, quartz, and others) produce a voltage when deformed by an applied pressure. Piezoelectricity also results in production of a pressure when these materials are deformed by an applied voltage.

Single-element transducers (other types are discussed in Section 4.5) are in the form of **discs** (Figure 4.1). When an electrical voltage is applied to the faces, the thickness of the disc increases or decreases depending on the polarity of the voltage. The term **transducer element** (also called piezoelectric element or active element) refers to the piece of piezoelectric material that converts electricity to ultrasound and vice versa. The element with its associated case and damping and matching materials (discussed later in this section) is called the **transducer assembly** or **probe** (Figure 4.2). Both the transducer element and the transducer assembly are commonly referred to as the transducer. Typical diagnostic ultrasound transducer elements are 3–20 mm in diameter and 0.2–3 mm thick.

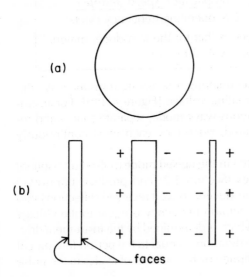

Figure 4.1. Disc transducer element. (a) Front view. (b) Side view with no voltage applied to faces (normal thickness), voltage applied (increased thickness), and voltage of opposite polarity applied (decreased thickness).

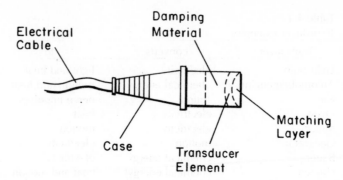

Figure 4.2. Transducer assembly or probe. The damping material reduces pulse duration, thus improving longitudinal resolution. The matching layer increases sound transmission into the tissues. The transducer element is usually curved for focusing (Section 4.4), but is sometimes flat (unfocused).

Source transducers operated in the **continuous mode (continuous wave mode)** are driven by a continuous alternating voltage (Section 5.6) and produce an alternating pressure that propagates as a sound wave [Figure 4.3(a)]. The frequency of the sound produced is equal to the frequency of the driving voltage. The operating frequency (sometimes called **resonant frequency**) of the transducer is its preferred frequency of operation. Operating frequency is determined by the propagation speed of the transducer material and the thickness of the transducer element.

$$\text{operating frequency (MHz)} = \frac{\text{propagation speed (mm/}\mu\text{s)}}{2 \times \text{thickness (mm)}}$$

$$\text{thickness (mm)} = \frac{\text{propagation speed (mm/}\mu\text{s)}}{2 \times \text{operating frequency (MHz)}}$$

where propagation speed is that for the transducer material (typically 4–6 mm/μs)

Continuous-wave sound encountering a receiving transducer is converted to a continuous alternating voltage [Figure 4.3(b)]. For instruments employing the continuous-wave mode, separate source and receiver transducers are required, since they each must continuously perform their function.

Source transducers operated in the **pulsed mode** (pulsed ultrasound) are driven by **voltage pulses** (Section 5.2) and produce ultrasound pulses (Figure 4.4). These transducers convert received reflections into voltage pulses. The pulse repetition frequency is equal to the voltage pulse repetition frequency, which is determined by the instrument driving the transducer. The pulse duration is equal to the period (reciprocal of operating frequency) multiplied by the number of cycles in the pulse

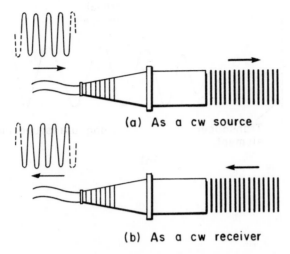

(a) As a cw source

(b) As a cw receiver

Figure 4.3. Transducer assembly operating in continuous wave (cw) mode. The device converts (a) a cw voltage into cw ultrasound or converts (b) received cw ultrasound into a cw voltage.

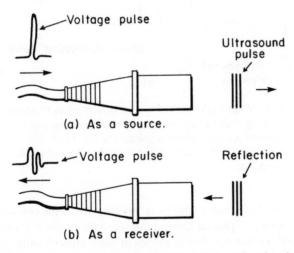

Voltage pulse

Ultrasound pulse

(a) As a source.

Voltage pulse

Reflection

(b) As a receiver.

Figure 4.4. Transducer assembly operating in pulsed mode. This device converts (a) electrical voltage pulses into ultrasound pulses and converts (b) received ultrasound pulses (reflections) into electrical voltage pulses.

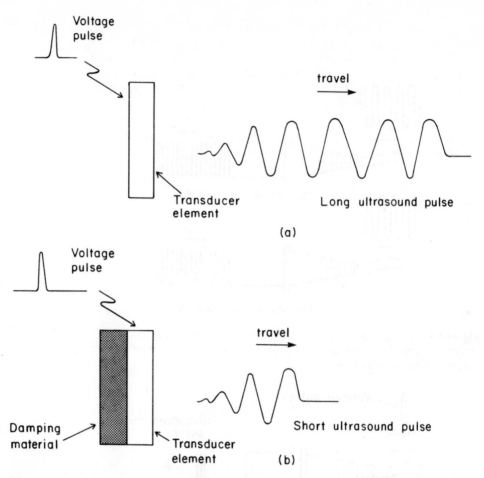

Figure 4.5. Without damping (a), a voltage pulse applied to a transducer element results in a long pulse of many cycles. With damping material on the rear face of the transducer element (b), application of a voltage pulse results in a short pulse of a few cycles. This figure shows each pulse traveling away from the transducer from left to right in space so that the right-hand end is the beginning or leading edge of the pulse.

(Section 2.3). Damping material (a mixture of metal powder and a plastic or epoxy) is placed behind the rear face of the transducer element to reduce the number of cycles in each pulse (Figure 4.5). This reduces pulse duration and spatial pulse length and thus results in improved longitudinal resolution. This method of damping is analogous to packing foam rubber around a bell that is rung by a tap with a hammer. The rubber reduces the time that the bell rings following the tap. It also reduces the loudness or intensity of the ringing. For ultrasound transducers, the damping material reduces the ultrasound amplitude and thus decreases the efficiency and sensitivity of the system (undesired effect). This is the price paid for reduced spatial pulse length (desired effect resulting in improved longitudinal resolution). Some damping may also be accomplished electrically within the instrument. Typically, pulses of two to six cycles are generated with diagnostic ultrasound transducers. Transducers that produce two- or three-cycle pulses are preferable because of improved longitudinal resolution.

A **matching layer** is commonly placed on the transducer face (Figure 4.2). This material has an impedance intermediate between those of the transducer element and the tissue. It reduces the reflection of ultrasound at the transducer element surface, improving sound transmission into the element. This is analogous to the coating layer on a camera lens that improves light transmission at the lens surface.

Because of the very low impedance of air, even a very thin layer of air between the transducer and the skin surface will reflect virtually all the sound, preventing any penetration into the tissue. For this reason, a coupling medium, usually an aqueous gel or mineral oil, is applied to the skin prior to transducer contact. This eliminates the air layer and permits the sound to pass into the tissue.

The materials from which most transducer elements are made become piezoelectric as part of the manufacturing process. They can lose their piezoelectric property if heated above the critical temperature (Curie temperature) of approximately 350°C. For this reason, transducer assemblies should not be autoclaved.

A transducer operating in the pulsed mode prefers to produce a frequency equal to its operating frequency (introduced earlier in this section). However, the ultrasound pulses produced contain frequencies in addition to this. The shorter the pulse (the fewer the number of cycles), the more frequencies that are present. The range of frequencies involved in a pulse is called its **bandwidth. Quality factor** (Q factor) relates bandwidth to operating frequency:

$$\text{quality factor} = \frac{\text{operating frequency (MHz)}}{\text{bandwidth (MHz)}}$$

Quality factor is unitless. The inclusion of damping material in the transducer assembly increases the bandwidth and decreases the quality factor.

Exercises

4.2.1. A transducer converts one form of _____ to another.

4.2.2. Ultrasound transducers convert _____ energy into _____ energy and vice versa.

4.2.3. Ultrasound transducers operate on the _____ principle.

4.2.4. Single-element transducers are in the form of _____.

4.2.5. The _____ of a transducer element changes when a voltage is applied to the faces.

4.2.6. The term transducer is often used to refer to either a transducer _____ or a transducer _____.

4.2.7. A transducer _____ is part of a transducer _____.

4.2.8. A continuously alternating voltage applied to a transducer produces _____ ultrasound.

4.2.9. Electrical voltage pulses applied to a transducer produce ultrasound _____.

4.2.10. Operating frequency _____ as transducer element thickness is increased.

4.2.11. Addition of damping material to a transducer reduces the number of _____ in the pulse, thus improving _____ _____. It increases the _____ and decreases the _____ _____.

4.2.12. Addition of damping material reduces the _____ and _____ of the diagnostic system.

4.2.13. Ultrasound transducers typically generate pulses of _____ to _____ cycles.

4.2.14. If the propagation speed of the transducer element material is 4 mm/μs, the thickness required for an operating frequency of 10 MHz is _____ mm.

4.2.15. If the propagation speed of the transducer element material is 6 mm/μs, the operating frequency for a thickness of 3 mm is _____ MHz.

4.2.16. The matching layer on the transducer surface reduces _____ caused by impedance difference.

4.2.17. A coupling medium on the skin surface eliminates reflection caused by _____.

4.2.18. Quality factor is given in
a. MHz
b. mm/μs
c. percent
d. all of the above
e. none of the above

4.2.19. Increasing the bandwidth increases the quality factor. True or false?

4.2.20. The range of _____ involved in an ultrasound pulse is called its bandwidth.

61

The ultrasound pulse generated by the (flat) disc transducer in Figure 4.1 is contained in a cylindrical shape, as shown in Figure 4.6. The spatial pulse length was discussed in Sections 2.3 and 4.2. We shall now discuss the beam diameter.

4.3 Sound Beams

A single-element (flat) disc transducer operating in the continuous-wave mode produces a sound beam with a beam diameter that varies according to distance from the transducer face as shown in Figure 4.7. The intensity is not uniform throughout the beam (Section 2.4). The beam diameter shown in Figure 4.7 approximates that portion of the sound produced that is greater than 4 percent of the spatial peak intensity. This particular value was chosen because it gives the simplest picture. The 6-dB beam diameter that is often used is narrower than that pictured in Figure 4.7. It includes that portion of the sound that is greater than 25 percent of the spatial peak intensity. Sometimes significant intensity travels out in some directions not included in the beam as pictured. These additional "beams" are called **side lobes.**

The region from the disc out to a distance of one near-zone length is called the **near zone**, near field, or Fresnel zone. Near-zone length (also called near-field length) is given by the following equations:

$$\text{near-zone length (mm)} = \frac{[\text{transducer diameter (mm)}]^2}{4 \times \text{wavelength (mm}}$$

For soft tissues:

$$\text{near-zone length (mm)} =$$

$$\frac{[\text{transducer diameter (mm)}]^2 \times \text{frequency (MHz)}}{6}$$

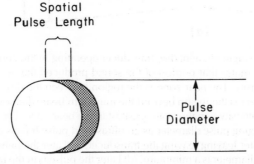

Spatial Pulse Length

Pulse Diameter

Figure 4.6. Ultrasound pulse generated by a single-element disc transducer driven by an electrical voltage pulse as in Figure 4.4. Pulse diameter is equal to beam diameter. This varies with distance from the transducer (Figure 4.7). Spatial pulse length is described in Figure 2.8.

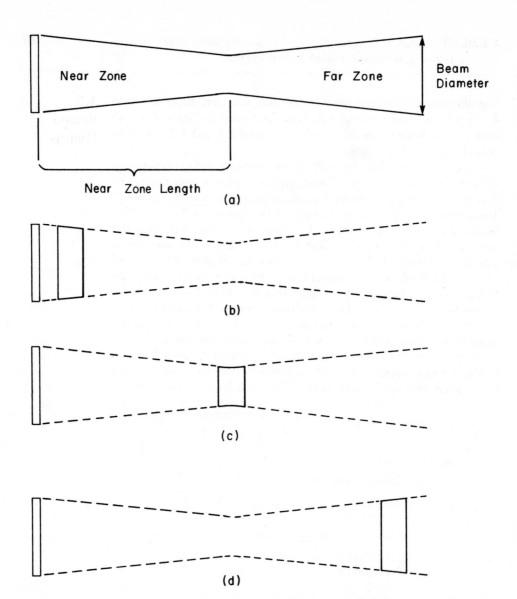

Figure 4.7. Beam diameter for a single-element disc transducer operating in the continuous-wave mode (a). This diameter approximates that portion of the sound produced that is greater than 4 percent of the spatial peak intensity. The near zone is the region between the disc and the minimum beam diameter. The far zone is the region beyond the minimum beam diameter. Intensity is not constant within the beam. Intensity variations are greatest in the near zone. The beam diameter in (a) approximates the changing pulse diameter as an ultrasound pulse travels away from the transducer. (b) A pulse shortly after leaving leaving the transducer. (c) Later the pulse is located at the near-zone length, where its diameter is a minimum. (d) Later the pulse is in the far field, where its diameter is increasing as it travels. This figure assumes a nonscattering nonrefracting medium such as water.

The region beyond a distance of one near-zone length is called the **far zone,** far field, or Fraunhofer zone.

The beam diameter depends on

1. wavelength (therefore frequency)
2. transducer diameter
3. distance from transducer

At a distance of one near-zone length from the transducer, the beam diameter is equal to one-half the transducer diameter. At a distance of two times the near-zone length, the beam diameter is equal to the transducer diameter. Beyond this distance, the beam diameter increases in proportion to distance.

In the near zone:

$$\text{beam diameter (mm)} = \left[\text{transducer diameter (mm)} - \frac{2 \times \text{wavelength (mm)} \times \text{distance (mm)}}{\text{transducer diameter (mm)}} \right]$$

In the far zone:

$$\text{beam diameter (mm)} = \frac{2 \times \text{wavelength (mm)} \times \text{distance (mm)}}{\text{transducer diameter (mm)}}$$

where distance is measured from the transducer face.

For soft tissues:

In the near zone:

$$\text{beam diameter (mm)} = \text{transducer diameter (mm)} - \left[\frac{3 \times \text{distance (mm)}}{\text{frequency (MHz)} \times \text{transducer diameter (mm)}} \right]$$

In the far zone:

$$\text{beam diameter (mm)} = \frac{3 \times \text{distance (mm)}}{\text{frequency (MHz)} \times \text{transducer diameter (mm)}}$$

where distance is measured from the transducer face.

The diameter of an ultrasound pulse (Figure 4.6) is equal to the beam diameter (Figure 4.7) for the distance from the transducer face at which the pulse is located at any given time. As the pulse travels through the near zone, its diameter decreases; as it travels through the far zone, its diameter increases.

Sound beams produced by disc transducers have beam areas given by the following equation:

$$\text{beam area (cm}^2\text{)} = 0.8 \times [\text{beam diameter (cm)}]^2$$

Example 4.3.1 For soft tissue and a 10-mm 5-MHz transducer, what are the beam diameters at 4, 8, 12, and 16 cm from the transducer? First find the near-zone length:

$$\text{near-zone length} = \frac{(\text{transducer diameter})^2 \times \text{frequency}}{6}$$

$$= \frac{10^2 \times 5}{6} = 83 \text{ mm} = 8.3 \text{ cm}$$

Distances of 4 and 8 cm are therefore in the near zone.

$$\text{beam diameter} = \text{transducer diameter} - \left[\frac{3 \times \text{distance}}{\text{frequency} \times \text{transducer diameter}}\right]$$

$$= 10 - \frac{3 \times 40}{5 \times 10} = 7.6 \text{ mm at 4 cm}$$

$$\text{beam diameter} = 10 - \frac{3 \times 80}{5 \times 10} = 5.2 \text{ mm at 8 cm}$$

Distances of 12 and 16 cm are in the far zone.

$$\text{beam diameter} = \frac{3 \times \text{distance}}{\text{frequency} \times \text{transducer diameter}}$$

$$= \frac{3 \times 120}{5 \times 10} = 7.2 \text{ mm at 12 cm}$$

$$\text{beam diameter} = \frac{3 \times 160}{5 \times 10} = 9.6 \text{ mm at 16 cm}$$

We see from this example that in the near zone, the beam diameter decreases with increasing distance from the transducer. In the far zone,

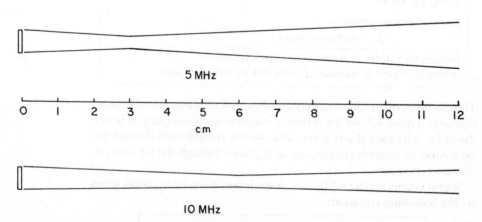

Figure 4.8. Beams for 6-mm diameter disc transducers of two frequencies. Higher frequency produces smaller beam diameter and longer near-zone length.

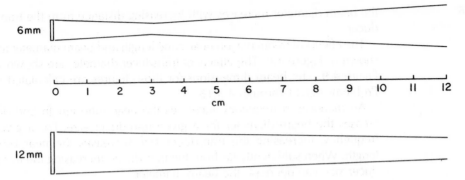

Figure 4.9. Beams for 5-MHz disc transducers of two diameters. The larger transducer produces the larger near-zone length. The right-hand portion of the figure shows that a smaller transducer can produce a larger-diameter beam.

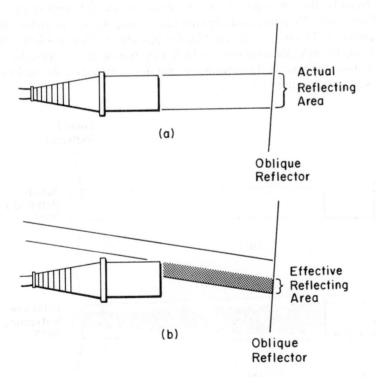

Figure 4.10. Oblique reflection. (a) Incident sound on reflecting area. (b) Reflected sound from reflecting area. Only part of this reflected sound (shaded portion) returns to the transducer from the effective reflecting area. The remainder misses the transducer and continues on. The effective reflecting area is smaller than the actual reflecting area. For simplicity, the beam shape shown in Figure 4.7 is ignored here.

the beam diameter increases with increasing distance from the transducer.

The effects of frequency on near-zone length and beam diameter are shown in Figure 4.8. The effects of transducer diameter are shown in Figure 4.9. The beam dimensions for those figures are calculated in Problems 4.3.11 through 4.3.18.

An increase in frequency increases the near-zone length and decreases the beam diameter for a given transducer size. For a given frequency, increasing the transducer size increases the near-zone length. When sufficiently far from the transducer, increasing the transducer size can *decrease* the beam diameter.

Since diagnostic ultrasound is confined to beams, there are conditions in which part or all of the reflected sound may not return to the transducer and thus will be missed. Figures 4.10 and 4.11 show examples of simple situations with oblique incidence in which this occurs. The **effective reflecting area,** the area that reflects sound that is received by the transducer, is smaller than the actual reflecting area in these cases. Therefore, reflector orientation and shape may reduce the amount of beam area received by the transducer. This problem is reduced by reflector roughness, which adds backscatter to specular reflection. Increasing the frequency effectively increases the reflector roughness (Section 3.2).

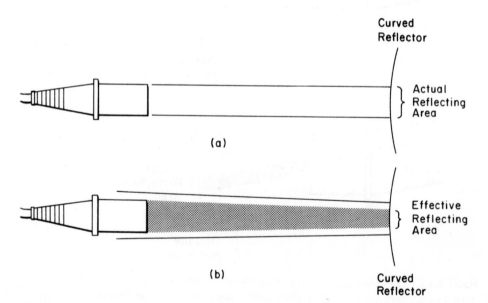

Figure 4.11. Curved reflector. (a) Incident sound on reflecting area. (b) Reflected sound from reflecting area. Only part of this reflected sound (shaded portion from the effective reflecting area) returns to the transducer. The remainder misses the transducer and continues on. The effective reflecting area is smaller than the actual reflecting area. For simplicity, the beam shape shown in Figure 4.7 is ignored here.

4.3.1. The beam diameter in Figure 4.7 includes that portion of the sound produced that is greater than _____ percent of the spatial peak intensity.

4.3.2. The beam is divided into two regions called the _____ zone and the _____ zone.

4.3.3. The dividing point between the two regions is at a distance from the transducer equal to one _____ length.

4.3.4. Beam diameter depends on _____, transducer _____, and _____ from the transducer.

4.3.5. Near-zone length is proportional to the square of the _____ _____ and inversely proportional to _____.

4.3.6. For a given medium (a given propagation speed), near-zone length is proportional to the square of the _____ _____ and to the _____.

4.3.7. At a distance of one near-zone length from the transducer, beam diameter is equal to _____ transducer diameter.

4.3.8. At a distance of _____ times the near-zone length, beam diameter is equal to transducer diameter.

4.3.9. In the near zone, beam diameter _____ as distance from the transducer increases.

4.3.10. In the far zone, beam diameter _____ as distance from the transducer increases.

4.3.11. For soft tissue and a 6-mm 5-MHz transducer, the near-zone length is _____ mm.

4.3.12. For Problem 4.3.11, the beam diameters at 15, 30, 60, and 120 mm from the transducer are _____, _____, _____, and _____ mm, respectively.

4.3.13. For soft tissue and a 6-mm 10-MHz transducer, the near-zone length is _____ mm.

4.3.14. For Problem 4.3.13, the beam diameters at 60, 120, and 180 mm from the transducer are _____, _____, and _____ mm, respectively.

4.3.15. In Problems 4.3.11 to 4.3.14, the higher-frequency transducer produces the _____ near-zone length and the _____ beam diameter at 120 mm from the transducer.

4.3.16. For soft tissue and a 12-mm 5-MHz transducer, the near-zone length is _____ mm.

4.3.17. For Problem 4.3.16, the beam diameters at 60, 120, 180, and 240 mm from the transducer are _____, _____, _____, and _____ mm, respectively.

4.3.18. In Problems 4.3.11, 4.3.12, 4.3.16, and 4.3.17, the larger transducer produces the _____ near-zone length and the _____ beam diameter at 120 mm from the transducer.

4.3.19. Doubling the transducer diameter _____ the near-zone length.

4.3.20. Doubling the frequency _____ the near-zone length.

4.3.21. If transducer diameter is doubled and frequency is halved, the near-zone length is _____.

**4.4
Lateral
Resolution
and
Focusing**

Lateral resolution is the minimum separation (in the direction perpendicular to the direction of sound travel or the direction of the beam) between two reflectors such that when the beam is scanned across them, two separate reflections are produced (Figure 4.12). **Lateral** resolution is equal to beam diameter.*

> lateral resolution (mm) = beam diameter (mm)

Recall that beam diameter varies with distance from the transducer, and therefore so does lateral resolution. If the lateral separation between two reflectors is greater than the beam diameter, two separate reflections are produced when the beam is scanned across them. Thus they are resolved, i.e., detected as separate reflectors.

*Like many statements in this book, this is a simplification of the actual situation that has been adopted for simplicity and brevity.

Figure 4.12. Lateral resolution. (a) Reflector separation (perpendicular to beam direction) is less than beam diameter. (b) Reflector separation is greater than beam diameter. (1) Sound travels from left to right and encounters the upper reflector (U), with part of the beam (shaded) being reflected back toward the source and the remainder continuing past the reflector. (2) The beam has been scanned down so that (a) it is partially reflected by both upper and lower (L) reflectors or so that (b) no reflection occurs, the beam completely passing between the reflectors. (3) The beam has been scanned down further so that part of it is reflected by the lower reflector, the remainder continuing past the reflector. (a) The scanning sequence (1)-(2)-(3) results in continual reflection from one or both of the reflectors. Separate reflections are not produced, and the reflectors are not resolved. (b) The scanning sequence (1)-(2)-(3) results in reflection from the upper reflector, then no reflection, then reflection from the lower reflector. Separate reflections are produced, and the reflectors are resolved.

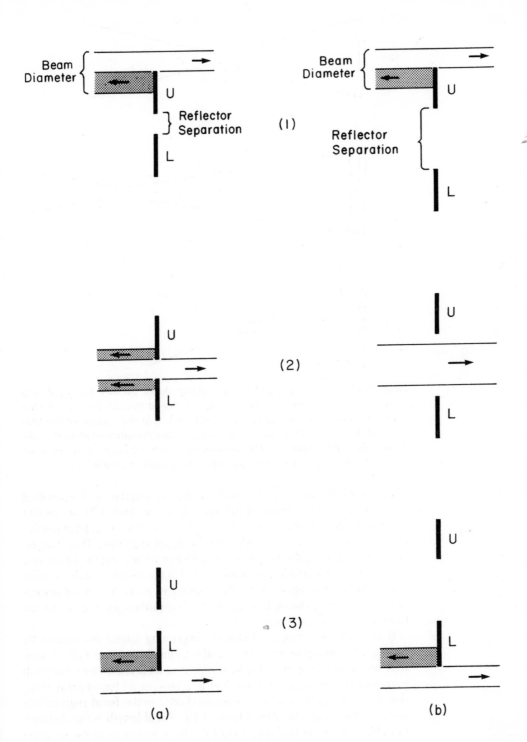

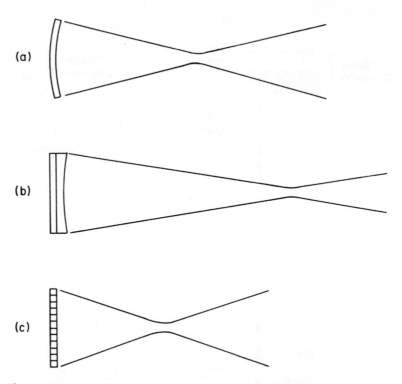

Figure 4.13. Sound focusing by (a) curved transducer, (b) lens, and (c) phased array. Lenses focus because the propagation speed through lenses is higher than that through tissues. Refraction (Section 3.3) at the surface of the lens forms the beam such that a focal region occurs. The operation of phased arrays is described in Section 4.5. The amount by which the beam diameter is reduced by focusing is described qualitatively as weak or strong focus.

Lateral resolution is also called transverse, angular, and azimuthal resolution. As with longitudinal resolution (Section 3.7), a smaller value indicates an improvement (finer detail is imaged). Lateral resolution may be improved by reducing the beam diameter. This may be done by increasing the frequency. Recall that increasing the frequency also improves longitudinal resolution, but at the expense of decreasing the depth of penetration. A smaller transducer improves lateral resolution near the transducer, but makes it worse farther out (e.g., at 10 cm from the transducer in Figure 4.9).

Beam diameter may be reduced (improving lateral resolution) by focusing the sound in a manner similar to the focusing of light. Sound may be focused (Figure 4.13) by employing a curved (rather than flat) transducer element, a curved reflector, a lens, or a phased **array** (Section 4.5). Lateral resolution is improved only in the **focal region;** it is worse in the region beyond (Figure 4.14). **Focal length** is the distance from the transducer to the center of the focal region or to the location of the spatial peak intensity. Its value is described qualitatively as short,

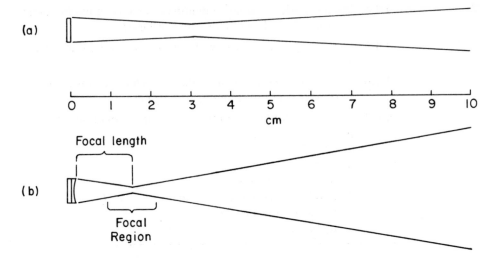

Figure 4.14. Beam diameter for 6-mm 5-MHz disc transducer of Figures 4.8 and 4.9 (a) without and (b) with focusing lens. Focusing in this case produces a minimum beam diameter half that for nonfocusing. However, beyond 2.5 cm from the transducer (outside the focal region), the focused beam diameter is greater than the unfocused.

medium, or long internal focus. The focal lengths associated with these terms vary with manufacturers. Internal focus refers to the use of a curved transducer element. The focal length cannot be greater than the near-zone length of the comparable (same transducer diameter and operating frequency) unfocused transducer. Some degree of focusing is common in diagnostic transducers. Diagnostic ultrasound transducers normally have better longitudinal resolution than lateral resolution, although the two may be comparable in the focal region for highly focused beams. Imaging *system* resolution is normally not as good as transducer resolution.

Exercises

4.4.1. Lateral resolution is the minimum _____ between two reflectors such that when a beam is scanned across them, two separate _____ are produced.

4.4.2. Lateral resolution is equal to _____ _____ .

4.4.3. Lateral resolution is also called (more than one correct answer)
   a. axial resolution
   b. longitudinal resolution
   c. angular resolution
   d. azimuthal resolution
   e. range resolution
   f. transverse resolution
   g. depth resolution

4.4.4. For a transducer of given diameter, increasing the frequency improves lateral resolution. True or false?

4.4.5. Lateral resolution varies with distance from the transducer. True or false?

4.4.6. For a given frequency, a smaller transducer always gives improved lateral resolution. True or false?

4.4.7. Lateral resolution is determined by (more than one correct answer)
   a. damping
   b. frequency
   c. transducer diameter
   d. number of cycles in the burst
   e. distance from transducer
   f. focusing

**4.5
Arrays**

Transducer arrays are transducer assemblies with more than one transducer element. The elements may be rectangular in shape and arranged in a line **(linear array)**, square in shape and arranged in rows and columns (two-dimensional or area array), or ring-shaped and arranged concentrically **(annular array)** (Figure 4.15).

A **linear switched array** (sometimes called a linear sequenced array or simply a linear array) is operated by applying voltage pulses to groups of elements in succession (Figure 4.16). Each group of elements acts like a larger transducer element in this case. The sound beam produced moves across the face of the transducer assembly and thus produces the same effect as **scanning** with a single-element transducer. However, such electronic scanning can be done in a more rapid and more consistent manner. If this electronic scanning is repeated rapidly enough, a **real-time** presentation of information can result (Section 5.5). This requires scanning across the transducer assembly several times per second.

A **linear phased array** (sometimes called a phased array) is operated by applying voltage pulses to all elements in the assembly as a complete group, but with small time differences, so that the resulting beam may be shaped and steered (Figure 4.17). If the same time differences are used each time the process is repeated, the same beam shape and direction will result repeatedly. However, the time differences may be changed with each successive repetition, so that the beam shape or direction can continually change. This can then result in sweeping of the beam (the beam direction changes with each pulse) and in dynamic focusing (the focal length changes with each pulse).

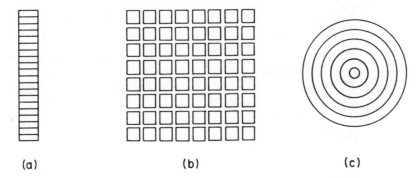

Figure 4.15. Front views of (a) linear array with 20 rectangular elements, (b) two-dimensional (area) array with 64 square elements, and (c) annular array with 6 elements.

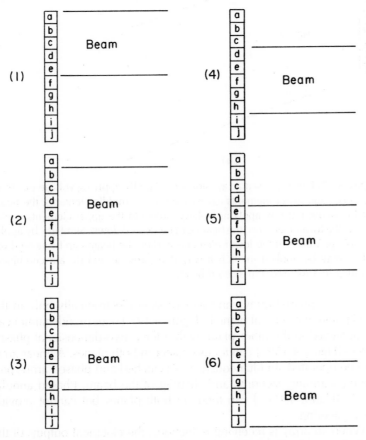

Figure 4.16. Linear switched array (side view). Voltage pulses are applied simultaneously to all elements in a group: (1) first to elements a through e as a group, (2) next to elements b through f, (3) next to elements c through g, and so on across the transducer assembly. Then the process is repeated.

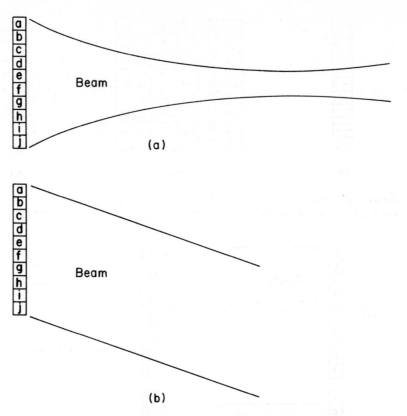

Figure 4.17. Linear phased array (side view). (a) By applying voltage pulses to the upper and lower elements earlier than to the middle elements, the beam can be focused. (b) By applying voltage pulses to the upper elements earlier than to the lower elements, the beam can be steered down. Similarly, by applying voltage pulses to the lower elements earlier, the beam can be steered up. Pulses may be applied in such a way that parts (a) and (b) are combined, resulting in a focused *and* steered beam.

A linear phased array can focus or steer electronically only in the scan plane (the vertical plane in Figure 4.17). Focus (nondynamic) can be achieved in the other plane with a lens. Two-dimensional phased arrays [Figure 4.15(b)] can focus or steer in both planes. A linear array can be operated simultaneously as a switched and phased array, providing scanning, steering, and shaping of the beam. Phased annular arrays [Figure 4.15(c)] can focus in both planes but cannot provide beam steering.

When an array is receiving reflections, the electrical outputs of the elements can be timed so that the array "listens" in a particular direction with a listening focus at a particular depth.

4.5.1. Transducer arrays are transducer assemblies with more than one transducer _____ .

4.5.2. Three types of arrays are _____ , _____ , and _____ .

4.5.3. Linear arrays are of two types according to how they are operated: linear _____ arrays and linear _____ arrays.

4.5.4. Match the following (answers may be used more than once):

a. A linear switched array can __*1*__ the beam.

b. A linear switched array cannot __*2*__ nor __*3*__ the beam.

1. scan
2. steer
3. shape

c. A linear phased array can __*2*__ and __*3*__ the beam.

d. A linear phased array can __*3*__ the beam but cannot __*1*__ nor __*2*__ the beam.

e. A linear switched and phased array can __*1*__, __*2*__, and __*3*__ the beam.

4.5.5. A linear array can scan, steer, or shape in _____ dimension(s).

4.5.6. A two-dimensional array can scan, steer, or shape in _____ dimension(s).

4.5.7. An annular array can shape in _____ dimension(s).

4.5.8. Match the following (answers may be used more than once):

a. linear switched array: _____

b. linear phased array: _____

c. two-dimensional phased array: _____

d. annular phased array: _____

1. Voltage pulses are applied in succession to groups of elements.
2. Voltage pulses are applied to all elements as a group, but with small time differences.

4.5.9. In Figure 4.17, if elements are pulsed in the order a, b, c, d, e, f, g, h, i, j, the resulting beam is
a. steered up   c. focused
b. steered down

4.5.10. In Figure 4.17, if elements are pulsed in the order j, i, h, g, f, e, d, c, b, a, the resulting beam is
a. steered up   c. focused
b. steered down

4.5.11. In Figure 4.17, if elements are pulsed in order a and j, b and i, c and h, d and g, e and f, the resulting beam is
a. steered up   c. focused
b. steered down

**4.6
Review**

Transducers convert energy from one form to another. Ultrasound transducers convert electrical energy to ultrasound energy and vice versa. They operate on the piezoelectricity principle. Transducers may be operated in continuous mode or pulsed mode. Pulsed transducers have damping material to shorten the spatial pulse length. Disc transducers produce sound in the form of beams with near and far zones. Lateral resolution is equal to beam diameter. Beam diameter may be reduced by focusing. Transducer arrays provide the ability to electronically scan, steer, and shape beams. If scanning or steering is repeated rapidly, real-time imaging can result.

Exercises

4.6.1. Match the following transducer assembly parts with their functions:
a. cable: _____
b. damping material: _____
c. piezoelectric element: _____
d. matching layer: _____

1. reduces reflection at transducer surface
2. converts voltage pulses to sound pulses
3. reduces pulse duration
4. conducts voltage pulses

4.6.2. Which of the following improve sound transmission from the transducer element into the tissue? (More than one correct answer.)
a. matching layer
b. Doppler effect
c. damping material
d. coupling medium
e. refraction

4.6.3. A transducer has thickness 0.4 mm, diameter 13 mm, and element material propagation speed 4 mm/μs. Calculate the following:

a. operating frequency:
_____ MHz

b. wavelength in soft tissue:
_____ mm

c. near-field length in soft tissue:
_____ mm

d. lateral resolution at 7 cm:
_____ mm

e. lateral resolution at 14 cm:
_____ mm

4.6.4. Lateral resolution is improved by

a. damping

b. pulsing

c. focusing

d. reflecting

e. absorbing

4.6.5. For an unfocused transducer, the best lateral resolution (minimum beam diameter) is _____ times the transducer diameter. This value of lateral resolution is found at a distance from the transducer face equal to the _____ length.

4.6.6. For a focused transducer, the best lateral resolution (minimum beam diameter) is found in the _____ region.

4.6.7. An unfocused 3.5-MHz 13-mm-diameter transducer will give a minimum beam diameter (best lateral resolution) of _____ mm.

4.6.8. An unfocused 3.5-MHz 13-mm-diameter transducer produces bursts of 3 cycles. The longitudinal resolution is _____ mm.

4.6.9. In Problems 4.6.7 and 4.6.8, longitudinal resolution is better than lateral resolution. True or false?

4.6.10. Longitudinal resolution is often not as good as lateral resolution in diagnostic ultrasound. True or false?

4.6.11. The two resolutions may be comparable in the _____ region of a highly focused beam.

4.6.12. Beam diameter may be reduced in the near zone by focusing. True or false?

4.6.13. Beam diameter may be reduced in the far zone by focusing. True or false?

4.6.14. Match each transducer characteristic with the sound beam characteristic it determines (answers may be used more than once):

a. element thickness: _____   1. longitudinal resolution
    and _____   2. lateral resolution
b. element diameter: _____   3. operating frequency
c. element shape (flat or curved): _____
d. damping: _____

4.6.15. The longitudinal resolution of a transducer can be improved most by
a. increasing the damping
b. increasing the diameter
c. decreasing the damping
d. decreasing the frequency
e. decreasing the diameter
f. attaching a Dopple

4.6.16. The principle on which ultrasound transducers operate is the
a. Doppler effect
b. acousto-optic effect
c. acoustoelectric effect
d. cause and effect
e. piezoelectric effect

4.6.17. Which of the following is *not* decreased by damping?
a. refraction
b. pulse duration
c. spatial pulse length
d. efficiency
e. sensitivity

4.6.18. Which three things determine beam diameter for a disc transducer?
a. pulse duration
b. frequency
c. disc diameter
d. distance from disc face
e. efficiency

Chapter 5

Instrumentation

In the preceding chapters we described how ultrasound is generated and how it interacts with tissues. The instrumentation that can detect and present the information resulting from this interaction will now be considered.

There are two basic ways (Figure 5.1) in which this information may be collected:

1. transmission
2. reflection

Transmission consists in ultrasound generation, propagation through tissues, and reception on the opposite side. It is analogous to receiving visual information from a photographic transparency by looking at the light that has passed through it.

Reflection consists of ultrasound generation, propagation, and reflection in tissues and reception of returning reflections. It is analogous to looking at the light that has reflected from the surface of a photographic print.

Transmission systems have been and are being studied for diagnostic ultrasound use. However, most diagnostic ultrasound systems in use today are the reflection (pulse-echo) type. These instruments detect three things: the strength, direction, and arrival time of reflections that occur in the tissues. Doppler instruments detect a fourth thing: the Doppler shift of these reflections.

This chapter will describe what the instruments do with the strength, direction, arrival time, and Doppler shift of received reflections.

5.1
Introduction

79

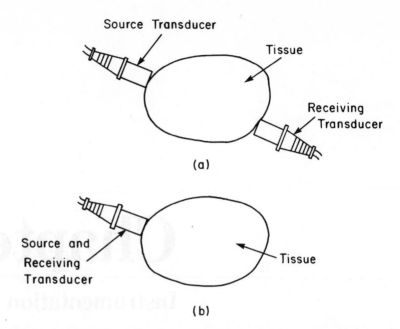

Source Transducer

Tissue

Receiving
Transducer

(a)

Source and
Receiving
Transducer

Tissue

(b)

Figure 5.1. Diagnostic ultrasound information collection methods. (a) Transmission. This method responds to attenuation and propagation speed encountered in the tissue. (b) Reflection. This method responds to reflection, attenuation, and propagation speed encountered in the tissue. For Doppler instrumentation it responds to Doppler shift.

5.2 Imaging System

Imaging systems produce a visual display from the electrical voltages received from the transducer. A diagram of the components of a pulse-echo imaging system is given in Figure 5.2. Several parameters that describe ultrasound were given in Chapters 2, 3, and 4. They are determined in this system as shown in Table 5.1.

The pulser is where the action originates. It produces electrical voltage pulses (Figure 5.3) that (1) drive the transducer, producing ultrasound pulses, and (2) tell the display when the ultrasound pulses are produced. The pulse repetition frequency of the pulser is the number of electrical pulses produced per second. It is typically 1000 Hz or 1 kHz. The ultrasound pulse repetition frequency is equal to the voltage pulse repetition frequency, since one ultrasound pulse is produced for each voltage pulse (Figure 5.4). Similarly, the ultrasound pulse repetition period is equal to the voltage pulse repetition period. The voltage pulse duration is less than the period of the cycles in the ultrasound pulses. To receive information for display at a rapid rate, it is necessary to use a high repetition frequency. However, repetition frequency must be limited in order to provide an unambiguous display of returning reflections. This will be described in Section 5.4.

Table 5.1
Determination of Ultrasound Parameters*

Ultrasound parameter	Determined by
Frequency	transducer
Period	transducer
Wavelength	transducer, tissue
Propagation speed	tissue
Pulse repetition frequency	pulser
Pulse repetition period	pulser
Pulse duration	transducer
Duty factor	pulser, transducer
Spatial pulse length	transducer, tissue
Longitudinal resolution	transducer, tissue
Amplitude	pulser, transducer, tissue
Intensity	pulser, transducer, tissue
Attenuation	transducer, tissue
Depth of penetration	transducer, tissue
Beam diameter	transducer, tissue
Lateral resolution	transducer tissue

*The ultrasound parameters described in Chapters 2, 3, and 4 are determined by imaging system components described in Chapters 4 and 5 (Figure 5.2). Overall imaging system longitudinal and lateral resolutions are also determined by the receiver and display.

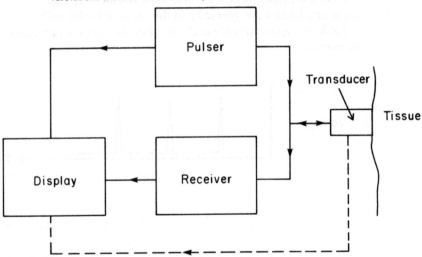

Figure 5.2. Components of a pulse-echo imaging system. The pulser produces electrical pulses (Figure 5.3) that drive the transducer. It also produces pulses that tell the display when the transducer has been driven. The transducer (acting as a source) produces an ultrasound pulse (Figure 5.4) for each electrical pulse applied. For each reflection received from the tissues, an electrical voltage is produced by the transducer (acting as a receiving transducer). These voltages go to the receiver, where they are processed to a form suitable for driving the display. For some display formats (Section 5.4), information on transducer position (location) and orientation (which way it is pointing) must be delivered (dash line) by electrical voltages to the display.

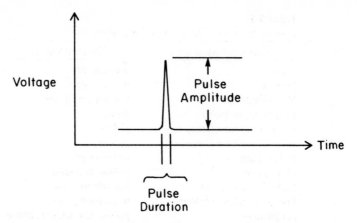

Figure 5.3. Electrical voltage pulse produced by the pulser and applied to the transducer. The transducer responds to the pulse by producing an ultrasound pulse (Figure 5.4).

The greater the pulse amplitude produced by the pulser, the greater will be the amplitude and intensity of the ultrasound pulses produced by the transducer. Ultrasound pulse amplitude and intensity depend also on the tissue impedance and the transducer efficiency. Electrical pulse amplitudes are generally in the range 20–600 volts.

Table 5.2 gives typical ranges for acoustic outputs of diagnostic instruments.

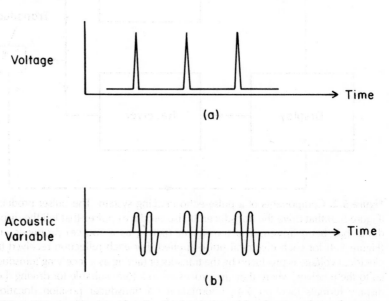

Figure 5.4. An ultrasound pulse (b) is produced by the transducer for every voltage pulse (a) applied.

Table 5.2

Typical Values for Acoustic Output Parameters of Diagnostic Ultrasound Imaging Instruments[6]

Parameter	Range
SATA intensity*	0.1–10 mW/cm²
SPTA intensity	0.01–200 mW/cm²
SPTP intensity	0.5–200 W/cm²
SP/SA factor	
Unfocused	2–3
Focused	5–200
Duty factor	0.001–0.003
Cycles per pulse	2–6
Pulse repetition frequency	0.5–3 kHz

*The lower limit of SPTA intensity is smaller than that for SATA intensity because SATA intensity was not measured on all units discussed by Carson et al.[6] An example comparing the various intensities is given in Section 2.4.

Exercises

5.2.1. The four primary components of a diagnostic ultrasound imaging system are the ___TRAN___, ___PULSER___, ___Receiver___, and ___Display___.

5.2.2. Match each component with its function:
a. pulser: __1__
b. transducer: _____
c. receiver: _____
d. display: _____

1. produces ultrasound pulses
2. processes voltages received from the transducer
3. receives processed electrical information from the receiver
4. produces electrical pulses that drive the transducer

5.2.3. Match these ultrasound parameters produced by an instrument with the components that determine them (answers may be used more than once):
a. frequency: __2__
b. period: __2__
c. wavelength: __2, 3__
d. propagation speed __3__
e. pulse repetition frequency: __1__
f. pulse repetition period: __1__

1. pulser
2. transducer
3. tissue

g. pulse duration: _____

h. duty factor: _____,

_____

i. spatial pulse length: _____,

_____

j. longitudinal resolution:

_____, _____

k. amplitude: _____,

_____, _____

l. intensity: _____, _____,

m. attenuation: _____,

_____

n. depth of penetration: _____, _____

o. beam diameter: _____,

_____

p. lateral resolution:

_____, _____

5.2.4. The ultrasound pulse repetition frequency is equal to the voltage _____ repetition frequency of the pulser.

5.2.5. Increased pulse amplitude produced by the pulser increases the _____ and _____ of ultrasound pulses produced by the transducer.

5.2.6. Match these acoustic parameters produced by diagnostic instruments with their typical values:

a. SATA intensity: _____   1. 50
b. SPTP intensity: _____   2. 0.002
c. SP/SA factor: _____   3. 1 mW/cm²
d. duty factor: _____   4. 3
e. cycles per pulse: _____   5. 10 W/cm²

5.3 Receiver

Voltages produced in the transducer by returning reflections are sent to the receiver for processing. The receiver performs the following functions:

1. **amplification**
2. **compensation**
3. **compression**
4. **demodulation**
5. **rejection**

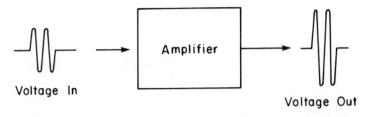

Voltage In   Voltage Out

Figure 5.5. Amplification increases voltage amplitude and electrical power.

Amplification consists in increasing the small voltages received from the transducer to larger ones suitable for processing and display (Figure 5.5). **Gain** is the ratio of output to input electrical power. The power ratio is equal to the square of the voltage ratio (across the same resistance); power ratio may be expressed in decibels (Appendix 4). For example, if input voltage amplitude to an **amplifier** is 2 mV and output voltage amplitude is 40 mV, the voltage ratio is 40/2 or 20. The power ratio is $(20)^2$ or 400. From Table A4.1 the power ratio or gain is found to be 26 dB. Receiver amplifiers usually have 60–100 dB of gain. Voltages applied to these amplifiers range from tens of microvolts to tens of millivolts.

Compensation (also called gain compensation, swept gain, time gain compensation, depth gain compensation) equalizes differences in received reflection amplitudes due to reflector depth. Reflectors with equal reflection coefficients (Section 3.2) will not result in equal amplitude reflections arriving at the transducer (Figure 5.6) if their travel distances are different (distances from the transducer to the reflectors are different). This is because attenuation depends on path length (Sections 2.5 and 3.5). It is desirable to display reflections from reflectors of equal reflection coefficients, sizes, and shapes in a similar way. Since these reflections may not arrive with the same amplitude, because of different path lengths, their amplitudes must be adjusted to compensate for path length differences. Larger path lengths result in later arrival times. Therefore, if voltages from reflections arriving later are amplified more than earlier ones, attenuation is compensated for. This is what compensation does (Figure 5.7).

Compression is the process of decreasing the difference between the smallest and largest amplitudes (Figure 5.8). The ratio of the largest power to the smallest power that the system can handle is called the **dynamic range.** It is expressed in decibels. For example, if the amplifier is insensitive to voltage amplitudes less than 0.1 mV and cannot properly handle voltage amplitudes greater than 100 mV, the ratio of voltages is 100/0.1 = 1000. The power ratio is equal to the square of the voltage ratio: $(1000)^2 = 1,000,000$. According to Table A4.1, the dynamic range of the amplifier is 60 dB. Although amplifiers and compensators have such a dynamic range, demodulators and displays do not. Their dynamic range is around 20 dB. The largest power can be

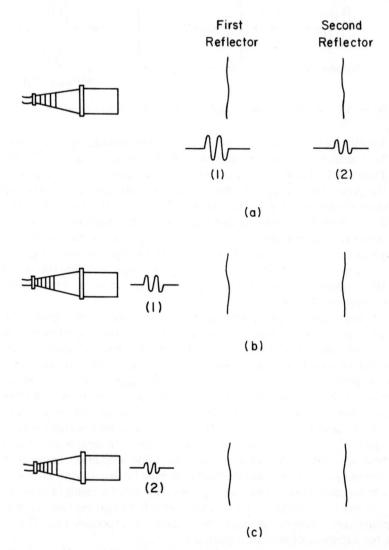

Figure 5.6. Two reflectors with equal reflection coefficients but different distances from the transducer. (a) The reflected pulse at the second reflector is weaker because the incident pulse has to travel farther to get to the second reflector, thus experiencing more attenuation. (b) The reflection from the first reflector arrives at the transducer. It is weaker than it was in (a) because of attenuation on the return trip. (c) The reflection from the second reflector arrives at the transducer later and weaker than the first one did. This is because of the longer path to the second reflector.

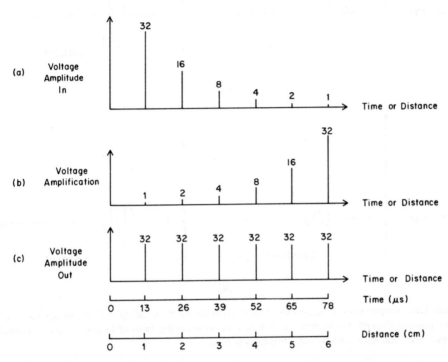

Figure 5.7. Compensation of attenuation by varying amplification. The time scale represents arrival time of reflections. The distance scale represents the distance from the transducer to the reflectors. (a) Arriving reflections produce different voltage amplitudes because of attenuation. All reflections are assumed here to have come from reflectors with equal reflection coefficients. Each reflection arrives 13 μs after the previous one, and thus for soft tissue each reflector is 1 cm farther from the transducer (Problem 3.6.6). Each reflection produces a voltage amplitude one-half that of the previous one. (b) Amplification must compensate for this by doubling as each 13 μs of time passes during the arrival of the reflections. Each arriving voltage amplitude (a) times the gain or amplification (b) existing at the time the voltage arrives at the amplifier equals the voltage amplitude out of the amplifier (c). Following this process, all the voltages are equalized. This is the case where all reflections result from equal reflection coefficients. If reflection coefficients of the various reflectors are different, the resulting voltage amplitudes, even after compensation, will be different. We would not want to normalize these differences and thus lose that information.

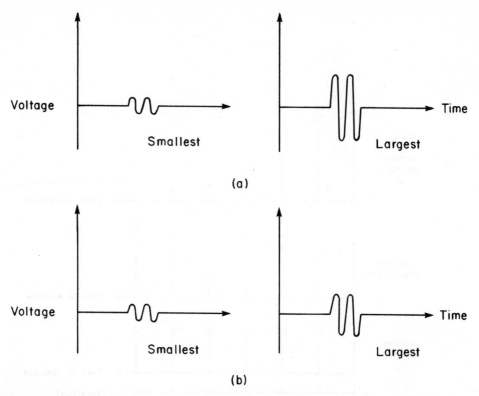

Figure 5.8. Compression decreases the difference between the smallest and largest voltage amplitudes passing through the system. (a) Before compression the ratio of largest to smallest amplitudes is five. (b) After compression the ratio is three.

only 100 times the smallest. Thus the largest voltage amplitude can be only 10 times the smallest. A compressor would have to compress the voltage ratio of 1000 in our example to a voltage ratio of 10. The most severe limitation on dynamic range is in photography of the display.

Demodulation (sometimes called detection or envelope detection) is the process of converting the voltages delivered to the receiver from one form to another (Figure 5.9). This is done by rectification and smoothing (Figure 5.10).

Rejection (sometimes called suppression or threshold) eliminates the smaller-amplitude voltage pulses produced by weaker reflections (Figure 5.11).

Figure 5.12 summarizes the five receiver functions discussed. The amplification (gain), compensation, and rejection functions are normally operator-adjustable; demodulation and compression are not.

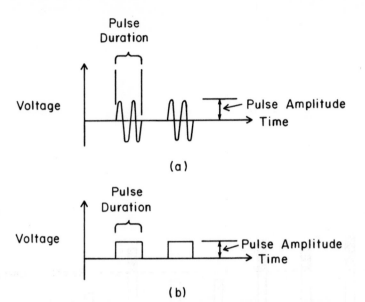

(a)

(b)

Figure 5.9. Demodulation is the conversion of pulses (a) to another form (b). Pulse amplitudes in (a) and (b) are proportional to each other. Pulse durations in (a) and (b) are equal to each other.

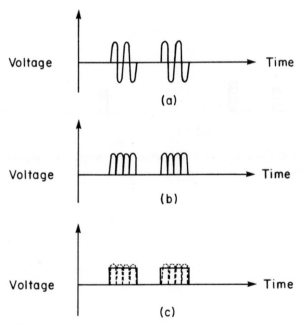

(a)

(b)

(c)

Figure 5.10. Rectification (b) and smoothing (c) of pulses (a) results in demodulation.

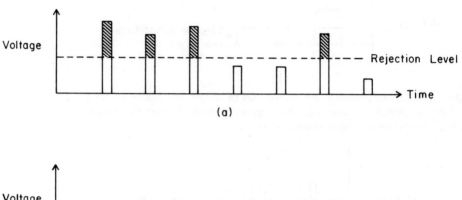

(a)

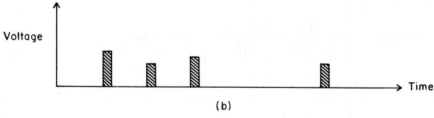

(b)

Figure 5.11. Rejection eliminates voltage pulses with amplitudes below the rejection level. (a) Before rejection. (b) After rejection.

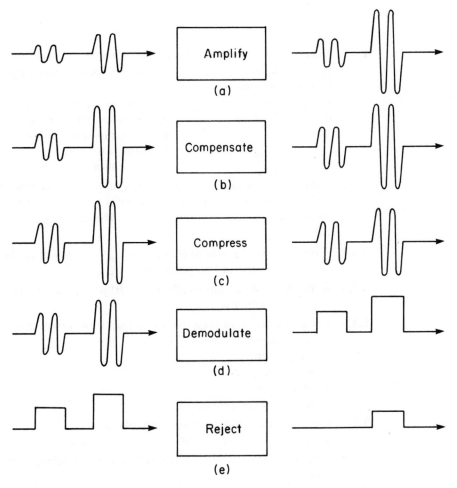

Figure 5.12. Five functions a receiver performs. The larger-amplitude pulse arrives first. (a) Both pulses are amplified, doubling their amplitudes in this example. (b) The latter (weaker) pulse is amplified more. (c) The difference between the pulse amplitudes is reduced. (d) The pulses are converted to another form. (e) The weaker pulse is rejected because it is not above the rejection level.

5.3.1. Five functions performed by the receiver are

_____, _____,

_____, _____, and

_____.

5.3.2. Match the following functions with what they accomplish:
a. amplification: _____   1. converts pulses from one
b. compensation: _____   form to another
c. compression: _____   2. increases all amplitudes
d. demodulation: _____   3. decreases dynamic range
e. rejection: _____   4. eliminates some pulses
5. corrects for tissue
   attenuation

5.3.3. Input voltage to an amplifier is 1 mV, and output voltage is 100 mV. The voltage amplification ratio is _____. The power ratio is _____. The gain is _____ dB.

5.3.4. A receiver with a gain of 60 dB has 1 μW of power applied to the input. The output power is _____ watt(s).

5.3.5. A receiver with a gain of 60 dB has 10 μV applied to the input. The output is _____ mV.

5.3.6. Compensation is also called (more than one correct answer)
a. swept beam
b. swept gain
c. refraction
d. diffraction
e. time gain compensation

5.3.7. Compensation takes into account reflector _____ or _____.

5.3.8. Compensation amplifies pulses differently, according to their arrival _____.

5.3.9. Compression decreases the _____ range to a range that the _____ and _____ can handle.

5.3.10. If a demodulator has a dynamic range of 20 dB and the smallest voltage it can handle is 200 mV, the largest voltage it can handle is _____ V.

5.3.11. Demodulation converts _____ or _____ from one form to another.

5.3.12. Rejection eliminates higher-amplitude pulses. True or false?

5.3.13. Another name for rejection is
   a. threshold
   b. depth gain compensation
   c. swept gain
   d. compression
   e. demodulation

There are several ways in which the pulses delivered from the receiver to the display may be presented. Those in common use are the following:

5.4 Display

1. **A mode**
2. **M mode**
3. **B mode**

The display device used in each case is a **cathode-ray tube**. This tube produces a sharply focused beam of electrons that produces a bright spot on the phosphor-coated front face (screen) of the tube (Figure 5.13). This spot can be moved across or up and down the face by applying voltages to the deflection plates (Figure 5.14). If the voltage applied to the horizontal deflection plates is properly varied, the spot can be made to move across the face at a constant speed. At the completion of this motion (i.e., when a **scan line** is completed), the spot can be made to jump rapidly back to the starting point on the left side of the face.

A-mode (amplitude-mode) operation causes a vertical deflection of the spot each time a pulse is delivered from the receiver (i.e., each time a reflection is received by the transducer). The horizontal position of the vertical deflection (Figure 5.15) is determined by pulse travel time (and thus by reflector distance). The vertical deflection amplitude is determined by the received reflection amplitude and by the amplification, compensation, compression, and rejection of the receiver. The A mode is commonly used in brain studies and in setting up M-mode presentations.

M-mode (motion-mode) operation causes a brightening of the spot, rather than a deflection, each time a reflection is received (Figure 5.16). In addition, each horizontal line is traced out slightly above the previous one. Back-and-forth motion of the reflector is seen as back-and-forth motion of the vertical deflection in the A mode or the bright spot in the M mode. The vertical movement of the M-mode display causes the motion of the reflector to be traced out. The M mode is commonly used in heart studies.

B-mode (brightness-mode) operation causes a brightening of the spot, as in the M mode. However, the scan lines are not horizontal as in the A and M modes. The starting point and direction of motion

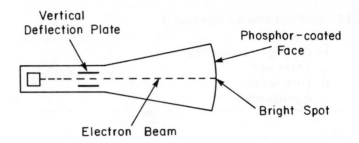

Vertical
Deflection Plate

Phosphor-coated
Face

Electron Beam

Bright Spot

Figure 5.13. Cathode-ray tube (side view). The electron beam produces a bright spot where it strikes the phosphor-coated face of the tube. There is a set of horizontal deflection plates that is not shown.

across the face are determined in the B mode by the position and orientation of the transducer (Figure 5.17). An image (**B scan**) of the object scanned may be built up on the face of the tube as the transducer is moved through many locations and orientations (Figure 5.18). Some means of storing the bright spots as the image is built up must be provided. This will be discussed later in this section. The B scan is an image that is a cross section of the object through the scanning plane, as if the sound beam were cutting a section through the object (a tomogram).

Another display mode, **C mode**, is not in common use. C-mode operation causes a brightening of the spot, as in the M and B modes. However, the scan lines are not traced out in the direction in which the transducer points as in the B mode. In the C mode the spot is positioned on the tube face in accordance with transducer location (Figure 5.19). If a reflection is received while the transducer is in a particular location, the spot is brightened. A cross-section image is produced by responding only to reflections from a specific distance or depth. This is accomplished by **gating** the receiver. Gating is the process of accepting only reflections that arrive at a certain time after the transducer produces a pulse. According to the range equation (Section 3.6), a given time corresponds to a given depth or distance. A C-mode image (**C scan**) is built up by scanning the transducer over a surface in two dimensions and storing bright spots at each position where reflections from the specified depth are received (Figure 5.20). The C scan is an image that is a cross section of the object parallel to the surface and at a depth selected by gating.

In all of the operating modes we have discussed it is assumed that for each pulse all reflections are received before the next pulse is sent out. If this were not the case, ambiguity could result (Figure 5.21). The maximum depth to be imaged by an instrument determines its maximum pulse repetition frequency. The relationship between pulse repetition frequency and maximum imaging depth in soft tissue is as follows:

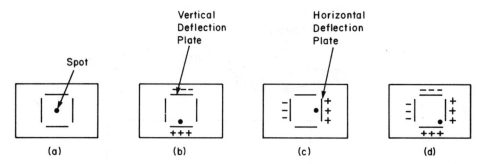

Figure 5.14. Spot deflection on the face of a cathode-ray tube (front view). (a) No voltage is applied to deflection plates; the spot is centered. (b) Voltage is applied to vertical deflection plates; the spot is deflected down. Increasing the voltage increases the deflection. If applied voltage were reversed, the spot would be deflected up. (c) Voltage is applied to horizontal deflection plates; the spot is deflected to the right. (d) Voltage is applied to both sets of plates; the spot is deflected down and to the right.

$$\text{pulse repetition frequency (kHz)} = \frac{77}{\text{maximum depth (cm)}}$$

$$\text{maximum depth (cm)} = \frac{77}{\text{pulse repetition frequency (kHz)}}$$

For many years diagnostic ultrasound displays used cathode-ray storage tubes that could not display various brightnesses. The amplitude of the pulse delivered by the receiver had little effect on the brightness of the spot displayed. The bright spots either were there or were not there. This is referred to as **bistable display** (on or off). In common use now is **gray-scale display,** in which several values of brightness may be stored and displayed. These displays produce B-scan presentations in which brightness is determined by received reflection amplitude. Higher-amplitude reflections may be presented as brighter spots or as darker spots. In some instruments either display method may be chosen.

The **scan converter** is a device that has made stored gray-scale displays possible. It stores the gray-scale image and allows it to be displayed on a television monitor. Gray-scale presentation of reflections preserves some of their dynamic range. Scan converters are capable of storing a greater dynamic range of brightness than the eye can handle. However, photography of displayed images usually limits the dynamic range to less than that of the eye.

M-mode display is usually recorded by a strip-chart recorder. B-mode displays are usually recorded by photography. Real-time displays (Section 5.5) are recorded on videotape.

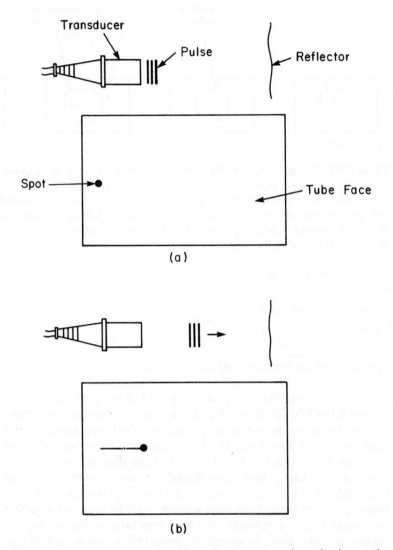

Figure 5.15. A-mode presentation of a reflection. (a) As the pulse leaves the transducer, the spot on the face of the cathode-ray tube begins to move to the right. (b) As the pulse moves toward the reflector, the spot continues to move to the right. (c) When the pulse is reflected, the spot has moved across the face an amount corresponding to half the transducer–reflector separation. (d) The spot continues to move to the right as the reflection moves toward the transducer. (e) When the reflection arrives at the transducer, an electrical pulse is delivered to the receiver, which delivers an electrical pulse to the display. This is applied to vertical deflection plates, causing the spot to deflect up at a horizontal position corresponding to the transducer–reflector separation. This process is repeated each time a pulse is delivered from the pulser to the transducer.

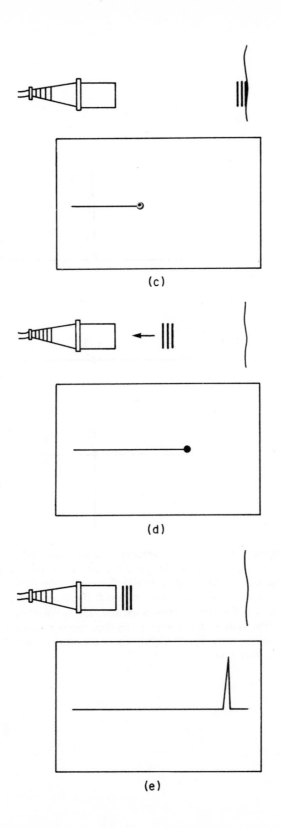

(c)

(d)

(e)

97

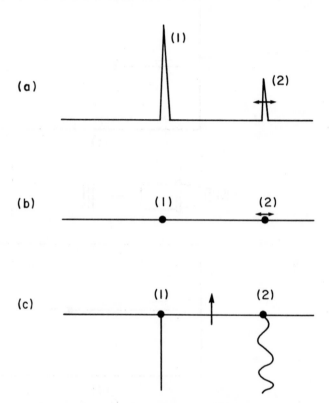

Figure 5.16. M-mode presentation of a reflection. Reflection 1 is produced at a stationary reflector. Reflection 2 is produced at a deeper reflector that is moving back and forth. (a) Vertical deflection 2 in the A mode moves left and right as the reflector moves closer to and farther from the transducer. (b) The bright spot 2 in the M mode moves left and right as the reflector moves closer to and farther from the transducer. (c) As the process is repeated and each horizontal scan line is positioned slightly above the previous one, the motion of reflector 2 is traced out.

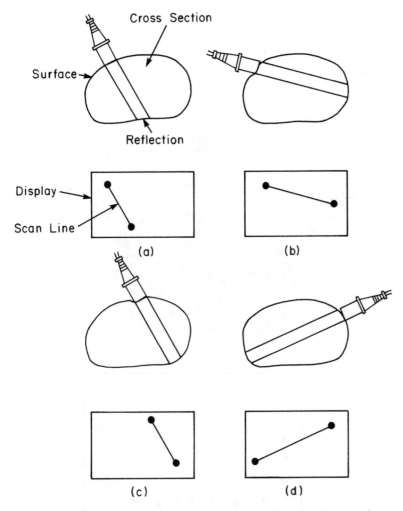

Figure 5.17. B-mode presentation of a reflection. (a) The transducer is shown in one location pointing in one direction. The reflection produces a bright spot on the display, as shown. (b) The transducer is in the same location as in (a), but it is pointing in another direction. The starting point for the scan line on the display is the same as in (a), but the line points in a different direction (the direction in which the transducer is pointing). (c) The transducer is in a location different from its locations in (a) and (b), but it is pointing in a direction parallel to that in (a). (d) The transducer is in the same location as in (c), but it is pointed in a different direction. By placing the transducer in many locations and orientations, a complete image (B scan) of the object scanned is built up on the display (Figure 5.18).

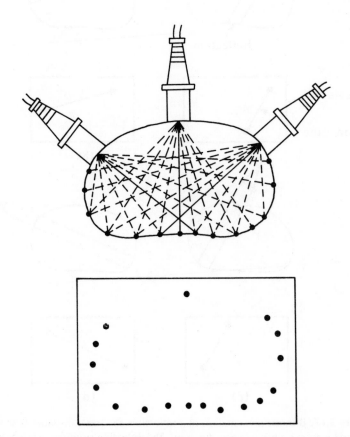

Figure 5.18. Building up a B-mode image (B scan) by moving the transducer through many locations and orientations.

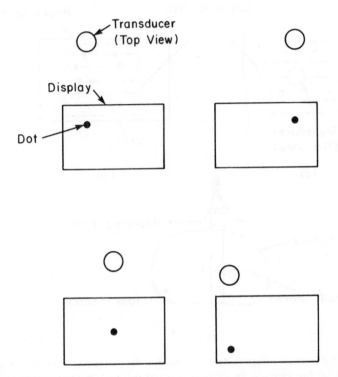

Figure 5.19. In the C mode the spot is positioned on the display in accordance with the location of the transducer. Various transducer positions and spot locations are shown.

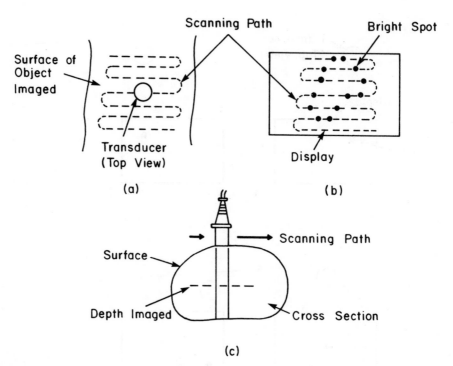

Figure 5.20. Building up a C-mode image (C scan) by moving the transducer over the surface of the object to be imaged. (a) Top view. As the transducer is moved, the spot moves on the display (b) and records bright spots where reflections return from the specified depth. (c) Cross-sectional view. Reflections are displayed from a given depth by gating the receiver according to the range equation.

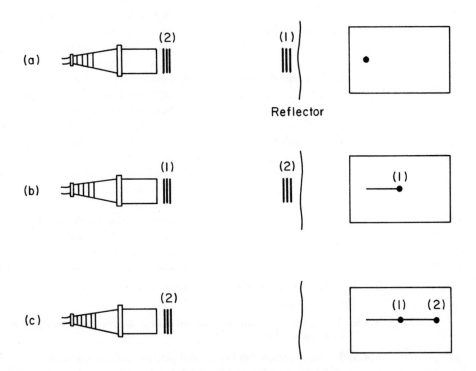

Figure 5.21. Ambiguity caused by sending out a pulse before a reflection from the previous pulse is received. (a) A pulse (2) is sent out just as a previous pulse (1) is reflected. The spot begins to move across the display. The first reflection arrives at the transducer when the second pulse reflects. (c) The second reflection arrives at the transducer, putting a bright spot (2) on the display at the position corresponding to the reflector. The spot (1) in the center of the display resulting from the arrival of the earlier pulse indicates a reflector at a location where there is none.

Exercises

5.4.1. The common methods of image presentation are called
_____ mode, _____ mode, and _____ mode.

5.4.2. Match the following display modes with appropriate
statements (answers may be used more than once):

a. A mode: _____,
_____

b. B mode (B scan):
_____, _____,
_____, _____

c. C mode (C scan):
_____, _____,
_____, _____,
_____

d. M mode: _____,
_____, _____

1. cross-sectional display
2. dot is deflected by return
   of a reflection
3. dot is brightened by return
   of a reflection
4. image of a section is
   parallel to surface scanned
5. vertical axis of display
   corresponds to time
6. dot moves with transducer
   position
7. scan lines move with
   transducer position and
   orientation
8. requires the transducer to
   be moved or scanned to
   develop the image
9. gives a one-dimensional display

5.4.3. The display device used in each mode is a
_____ tube.

5.4.4. The spot on a cathode-ray tube may be moved by applying
voltage to the _____ plates.

5.4.5. In the A mode the horizontal position of the vertical
deflection is determined by burst travel
_____ and thus by reflector
_____.

5.4.6. In the A mode a vertical deflection nearer the left-hand side
of the tube face results from a reflector that is nearer the
transducer. True or false?

5.4.7. The _____ mode is used for studying the motion of a
reflector.

5.4.8. To position a bright spot on the display in the B mode, the
instrument uses the arrival _____ of the
reflection and must assume a value for
_____ _____ in tissue.

5.4.9. The C scan presents a cross section at a
_____ chosen by gating the receiver.

5.4.10. The B scan presents a cross section through the
_____ plane.

5.4.11. The maximum permissible pulse repetition frequency that
will unambiguously image to a maximum depth of 30 cm
is _____ kHz.

5.4.12. The maximum depth for unambiguous imaging with an
instrument having a pulse repetition frequency of 1 kHz is
_____ cm.

5.4.13. A display that preserves some of the reflection dynamic
range is called a _____ display.

5.4.14. The _____ _____ stores the
gray-scale image and allows it to be displayed on a
television monitor.

Section 5.4 described how A-mode and M-mode presentations occur
with the transducer held stationary. However, it was shown that producing the two-dimensional images of the B mode and C mode required scanning the transducer. With such a manual scanning process,
it is not possible to produce images rapidly enough to produce a display that continuously images moving structures (**real-time display**).

There are two ways in which a real-time B-mode display can be
produced:

1. mechanically scan (sweep the sound beam)
2. electronically scan using an array

The first method may be accomplished by rotating the transducer with
a drive motor or by rotating a reflector. The rotating part is immersed in
a coupling liquid within the transducer assembly. The sound beam is
thus swept at a rapid rate without movement of the entire transducer
assembly. The second method is accomplished with a linear switched
array or a linear phased array, as described in Section 4.5.

Each complete scan of the sound beam produces an image on the
display that is called a **frame.** Each frame is made of scan lines (one for
each time the transducer is pulsed). In Section 5.4 we described the
limitation placed on pulse repetition frequency by the maximum depth
to be imaged. In real-time scanning the pulse repetition frequency, the
number of lines per frame, and the number of frames per second
(**frame rate**) are related to one another:

**5.5
Real Time**

pulse repetition frequency (Hz) = lines per frame × frame rate

The relationship among lines per frame, frame rate, and maximum imaging depth in soft tissue is as follows:

maximum depth (cm) × lines per frame × frame rate = 77,000

For example, if the maximum imaging depth desired is 20 cm and the frame rate is 20 frames per second, there will be approximately 200 lines per frame. If it is desired to image at greater depth, either the frame rate or the lines per frame will have to be reduced.

There are two primary advantages to real-time imaging:

1. more rapid and more convenient acquisition of the desired image
2. two-dimensional imaging of the motion of moving structures

The first advantage derives from the fact that the display continuously changes as the transducer is moved over the body surface. The second derives from the fact that the display continuously changes as the structures move.

Exercises

5.5.1. The modes that show one-dimensional real-time images are the _____ mode and the _____ mode.

5.5.2. The modes that can show two-dimensional real-time images are the _____ mode and the _____ mode.

5.5.3. A real-time B-mode display may be produced by rapid _____ transducer scanning or by _____ scanning of a transducer array.

5.5.4. Each complete scan of the sound beam produces an image on the display that is called a _____.

5.5.5. The number of lines in each frame is equal to the number of times the transducer is _____ while the frame is produced (while the sound beam is scanned).

5.5.6. In real-time scanning the pulse repetition frequency is equal to the product of the number of _____ per frame and the _____ rate.

5.5.7. If the maximum depth imaged is 30 cm and the frame rate is 20 frames per second, there are _____ lines per frame.

5.5.8. The pulse repetition frequency in Problem 5.5.7 is _____ kHz.

5.5.9. If there are 200 lines per frame and 20 frames per second, can 25 cm of depth be imaged?

5.5.10. Real-time imaging permits imaging of the motion of moving structures, but it is not as convenient as conventional B-mode imaging for acquiring desired static images. True or false?

One piece of information not used by the instruments described in Section 5.2 is the Doppler shift (Section 3.4) of the received reflections.

Doppler systems respond to moving reflectors (usually blood cells in the circulation) by detecting Doppler shift. This information is converted to audible sound or to a visual display. Doppler systems are of two types:

1. the continuous-wave Doppler system, which normally produces audible sound output
2. the pulsed system, which normally produces audible sound and may have visual display as well

A diagram of the components of a continuous-wave Doppler system is given in Figure 5.22. The voltage generator produces 5–50 V at 2–10 MHz, and this is applied to the source transducer. The ultrasound frequency is determined by the voltage generator. It is set equal to the operating frequency of the transducer (Section 4.2). In the transducer assembly there is a separate receiving transducer that produces a voltage with a frequency equal to the frequency of the reflected ultrasound. If there is reflector motion, the reflected ultrasound and the ultrasound produced by the source transducer will have different frequencies. The receiver detects the difference between these two frequencies (the Doppler shift) and drives a loudspeaker at this difference frequency. The Doppler shift is typically one-thousandth of the source frequency, which puts it in the audible range.

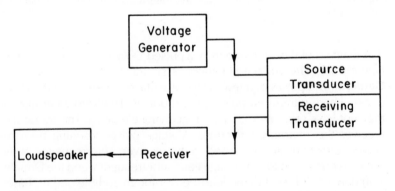

Figure 5.22. Continuous-wave Doppler system. The voltage generator produces a continuously alternating voltage that drives the source transducer. The receiving transducer produces a continuous voltage in response to reflections it continually receives. The receiver detects any difference in frequency between the voltages produced by the continuous-wave generator and by the receiving transducer. The Doppler shift produces a voltage that drives a loudspeaker in the audible range. The frequency of the audible sound is equal to the Doppler shift. It is proportional to the reflector speed and to the cosine of the angle between the sound propagation direction and the boundary motion (Section 3.4).

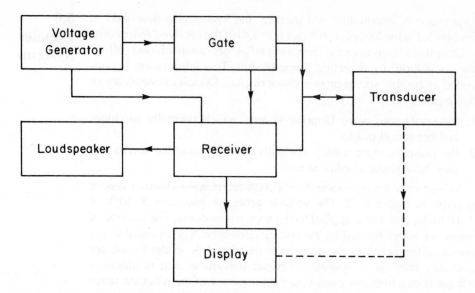

Figure 5.23. Pulsed Doppler system. The voltage generator produces a continuously alternating voltage. The gate converts this continuous voltage to voltage pulses that drive the transducer. This may be a single- or dual-element transducer. Received pulses are delivered to the receiver, where their frequency is compared to the generator frequency. The difference (Doppler shift) is sent to the loud-speaker. The receiver can select reflections from a given depth according to arrival time and thus give depth-motion information. A display may be included in this system, since it is capable of performing imaging also. The dotted line indicates transducer position and orientation information path to the display.

A diagram of the components of a pulsed Doppler system is given in Figure 5.23. The voltage generator is similar to that in Figure 5.22 **Gating** allows pulses of a few cycles of voltage to pass on to the transducer, where ultrasound pulses are produced. The transducer may or may not have separate source and receiving elements. The transducer receives the returning reflections. Voltage pulses resulting from received reflections are processed in the receiver. The frequency of the pulses is compared to the voltage generator frequency and the Doppler shift derived. It is sent to the loudspeaker for an audible output. Based on the arrival time of reflections, those coming from reflectors at a given depth may be selected; thus motion information may be obtained as a function of depth.

Doppler instrument SATA intensities range from 0.2 to 400 mW/cm^2.[6]

Exercises

5.6.1. Doppler systems convert _____ _____ information to audible sound or visual display.

5.6.2. A pulser similar to that used in imaging systems is used in Doppler systems. True or false?

5.6.3. Doppler system transducers may have _____ or _____ elements.

5.6.4. The receiver in a Doppler system compares the _____ of the voltage generator and the voltage from the receiving transducer.

5.6.5. The Doppler *shift* usually is not in the audible frequency range and must be converted by the receiver to a frequency that can be heard. True or false?

5.6.6. Doppler shift is determined by reflector _____ and by the cosine of an angle.

5.6.7. A component that pulsed Doppler systems have but continuous-wave Doppler systems do not have is the

_____.

5.6.8. A pulsed Doppler system may have as an output a visual

_____.

5.6.9. In a pulsed Doppler system, the pulse repetition frequency is determined by the _____, and the source ultrasound frequency is determined by the

_____ _____.

5.6.10. Pulsed Doppler systems can give motion information as a function of _____.

5.6.11. A typical SATA output intensity for a Doppler instrument is 10 mW/cm². True or false?

Artifacts in ultrasound imaging [3, 7–9] occur as structures that are one of the following:

1. not real
2. missing
3. of improper brightness
4. of improper shape
5. of improper size

5.7 Artifacts

Some artifacts are produced by improper equipment operation (e.g., improper transducer location and orientation information sent to the display) or settings (e.g., incorrect receiver compensation settings). Some are caused by improper scanning technique (e.g., allowing patient or organ movement during scanning). Others are inherent in the ultrasound diagnostic method and can occur even with proper equip-

Figure 5.24. Reverberation on the display. (1) First real reflector. (2) Second real reflector. (r) Reverberations. The separation betwen reverberations is the same as the separation between the real reflectors.

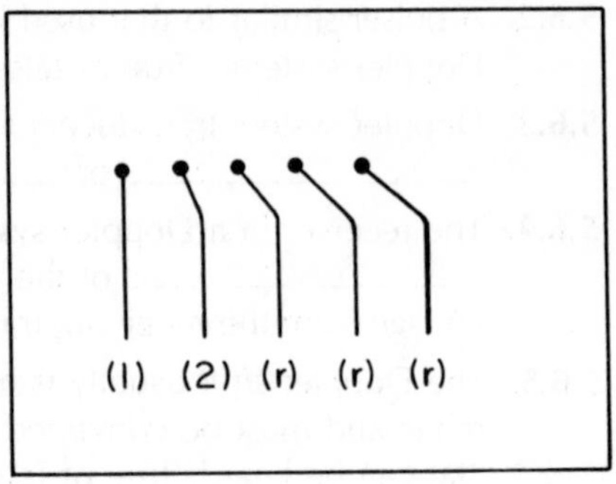

ment and technique. The factors that relate to these artifacts are the following:

1. reverberation
2. **shadowing**
3. **enhancement**
4. curved reflector
5. oblique reflector
6. propagation speed error
7. refraction and side lobes
8. **multipath**
9. resolution

Reverberation was discussed in Section 3.6. It results in reflectors that are not real being placed on the image. They will be placed behind the second real reflector (see Figure 3.7) at separation intervals equal to the separation between the first and second real reflectors (Figure 5.24). Each subsequent reflection will be weaker than prior ones. The first reflector in Figure 3.7 may be the transducer face.

Shadowing is the reduction in reflection amplitude from reflectors that lie behind a strongly reflecting or attenuating structure. Enhancement is the increase in reflection amplitude from reflectors that lie behind a weakly attenuating structure. Shadowing and enhancement result in reflectors being placed on the image with amplitudes that are too low and too high, respectively. A curved reflector can produce a reflection low in amplitude because some of the reflection is missed by the transducer (see Figure 4.11). Oblique reflection can produce a reflection low in amplitude, or the reflection may be completely missed by the transducer (see Figure 4.10).

Propagation speed error occurs when the assumed value for propagation speed in the range equation (Section 3.6) is incorrect. Diagnostic instrumentation assumes a speed of 1.54 mm/μs. If the propagation speed that exists over a path traveled is greater than 1.54 mm/μs, the calculated distance to the reflector is too small, and the display will

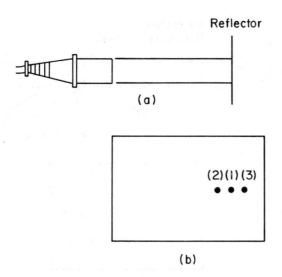

Reflector

(a)

(2)(1)(3)
● ● ●

(b)

Figure 5.25. Reflector position on the display (b) depends on the propagation speed over the traveled path (a). The reflector is actually in position 1. If the assumed propagation speed is too low, it will appear in position 2. If the assumed speed is too high, it will appear in position 3.

place the reflector too close to the transducer (Figure 5.25). If the actual speed is less than 1.54 mm/μs, the reflector will be displayed too far from the transducer (Figure 5.25).

Refraction (Section 3.3) can cause a reflector to be improperly positioned on the display (Figure 5.26). A similar occurrence can be caused by reflections from side lobes (Section 4.3). Refraction and propagation speed error can also cause a structure to be displayed with incorrect shape.

The term multipath describes the situation in which the paths to and from a reflector are different (Figure 5.27). Multipath results in improper reflector image positioning.

Resolution was discussed in Sections 3.7 and 4.4 in terms of separation of two reflectors (See Figures 3.8 and 4.12). If separation is not sufficient, two reflectors are seen as one (missing-reflector artifact). Resolution also increases the apparent size of a reflector on a display (Figure 5.28). The minimum displayed lateral and longitudinal dimensions will be the beam diameter and one-half the spatial pulse length, respectively.

Continuous-wave Doppler systems can give motion artifacts if reflectors with different motions are included in the sound beam (e.g., two blood vessels being viewed simultaneously). Pulsed Doppler systems help solve this problem by monitoring reflectors at selected distances or depths.

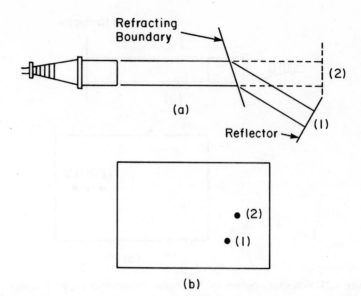

Figure 5.26. Improper positioning of reflector on the display (b) because of refraction (a). The system thinks the reflector is at position 2 because that is the direction in which the transducer is pointing. The reflector is actually at position 1.

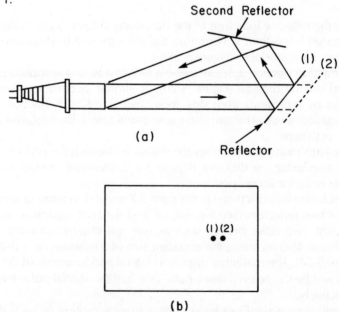

Figure 5.27. Improper positioning of reflector on the display (b) because of multipath (a). The system thinks that the reflector is at position 2 because of the increased round-trip travel time required for a longer return path. The reflector is actually at position 1.

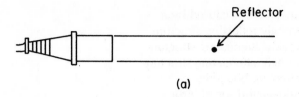

Reflector

(a)

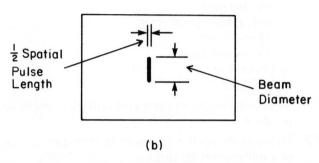

$\frac{1}{2}$ Spatial Pulse Length

Beam Diameter

(b)

Figure 5.28. A tiny reflector (a) is displayed (b) with the longitudinal dimension equal to one-half the spatial pulse length and the lateral dimension equal to the beam diameter.

5.7.1. Match these artifact causes with their results:

a. reverberation: _____
b. shadowing: _____,

_____

c. enhancement: _____
d. curved reflector: _____
e. oblique reflection: _____,

_____

f. propagation speed error:

_____, _____

g. refraction: _____, _____
h. multipath: _____
i. resolution: _____, _____

1. unreal structure displayed
2. structure missing on the display
3. structure displayed with improper brightness
4. improperly positioned structure
5. improperly shaped structure
6. structure of improper size

5.7.2. Reverberation results in added reflectors being imaged with equal _____.

5.7.3. In reverberation, subsequent reflections are _____ than previous ones.

5.7.4. Enhancement is caused by a
   a. strongly reflecting structure
   b. weakly attenuating structure
   c. strongly attenuating structure
   d. refracting boundary
   e. propagation speed error

5.7.5. A reflector may be missing from the display because of
   a. reverberation
   b. propagation speed error
   c. enhancement
   d. oblique reflection
   e. Doppler shift
   f. Snell's law

5.7.6. Shadowing results in decreased reflection amplitudes. True or false?

5.7.7. Propagation speed error results in improper _____ position of a reflector on the display.
   a. lateral
   b. longitudinal

5.7.8. If the propagation speed in a soft-tissue path is 1.60 mm/μs, a diagnostic instrument assumes a propagation speed too _____ and will show reflectors too _____ the transducer.
   a. high, close to
   b. high, far from
   c. low, close to
   d. low, far from

5.7.9. Multipath can occur with only one reflector. True or false?

5.7.10. The minimum displayed longitudinal dimension of a reflector is equal to
   a. beam diameter
   b. ½ × beam diameter
   c. 2 × beam diameter
   d. spatial pulse length
   e. ½ × spatial pulse length
   f. 2 × spatial pulse length

5.7.11. The minimum displayed lateral dimension of a reflector is approximately equal to
   a. beam diameter
   b. ½ × beam diameter
   c. 2 × beam diameter
   d. spatial pulse length
   e. ½ × spatial pulse length
   f. 2 × spatial pulse length

Most diagnostic ultrasound systems are of the reflection (pulse-echo) type. These use the direction, strength, and arrival time of received reflections to generate a one-dimensional A-mode or M-mode display or to generate a two-dimensional gray-scale B-mode or C-mode display. Sometimes motion detection and imaging are both performed by an instrument. Imaging systems consist of pulser, transducer, receiver, and display. Receivers amplify, compensate, compress, demodulate, and reject. Compensation equalizes differences in received reflection amplitudes caused by reflector depth. The A mode uses a deflection display. The M, B, and C modes use a brightness display. The M mode shows reflector motion in time. The B scan shows a cross section through the scanning plane. The C scan shows a cross section parallel to the surface and at a depth selected by gating. Maximum imaging depth is determined by pulse repetition frequency. Scan converters store gray-scale image information and permit display on a television monitor. Real-time displays are produced by rapid mechanically scanning transducers or electronically scanning arrays. Maximum depth imaged, lines per frame, and frame rate are related to one another. Doppler systems convert Doppler shift to an audible sound related to reflector motion. In pulsed Doppler systems, motion at selected depth is determined. Display artifacts may be caused by reverberation, shadowing, enhancement, curved reflector, oblique reflector, propagation speed error, refraction, side lobes, multipath, and resolution.

5.8 Review

Exercises

5.8.1. The reflector information that can be obtained from an M-mode display includes
   a. distance and motion pattern
   b. transducer frequency, reflection coefficient, and distance
   c. acoustic impedances, attenuation, and motion pattern
   d. size, orientation, and motion pattern

5.8.2. The compensation (swept gain, etc.) control serves to
   a. compensate for machine instability in the warmup time
   b. compensate for attenuation
   c. compensate for transducer aging and the ambient light in the examining area
   d. decrease patient examination time

5.8.3. A gray-scale display shows
   a. gray color on a white background
   b. reflections with one brightness level
   c. a white color on a gray background
   d. a range of reflection amplitudes

5.8.4. The dynamic range of an ultrasound system is best defined as
  a. the speed with which ultrasound examination can be performed
  b. the range over which the scanning arm can be manipulated while performing an examination
  c. the ratio of the maximum amplitude to the minimum amplitude or power that can be displayed
  d. the range of pulser voltages applied to the transducer

5.8.5. A real-time scan differs from a manual scan in that
  a. the real-time scan consists of many frames produced rapidly
  b. the manual scan image quality depends on how short a time the sonographer takes to make a scan
  c. the real-time scan is made only between 8 a.m. and 5 p.m.
  d. the real-time scan gives a gray-scale image, whereas the manual scan gives only an M-mode display.

5.8.6. Place the following in the order in which they are performed in a receiver:
  a. rejection
  b. amplification
  c. smoothing
  d. rectification
  e. compression
  f. compensation

5.8.7. Match the following (answers may be used more than once):
  a. A mode: _____, _____, _____
  b. B mode (B scan): _____, _____, _____
  c. C mode (C scan): _____, _____, _____
  d. M mode: _____, _____, _____

  1. one-dimensional
  2. two-dimensional
  3. real time
  4. real time or static
  5. deflection
  6. brightness

5.8.8. Continuous-wave sound is used in
  a. all imaging instruments
  b. some imaging instruments
  c. all Doppler instruments
  d. some Doppler instruments

5.8.9. If there were no attenuation in tissue, _____ would not be needed.
  a. rejection
  b. compression
  c. demodulation
  d. compensation

5.8.10. Match the following modes of display with the information that can be obtained:

a. A mode: _____, _____   1. reflector motion
b. M mode: _____, _____   2. reflector distance
c. static B mode: _____,   3. reflector shape
_____   4. reflector density
d. real-time B mode:

_____, _____, _____

e. static C mode: _____,

_____

f. real-time C mode: _____,

_____, _____

5.8.11. Transmission consists of ultrasound generation, propagation through tissues, and _____ on the opposite side.

5.8.12. Reflection consists of ultrasound generation, propagation and reflection in tissues, and reception of returning

_____.

5.8.13. Virtually all the diagnostic ultrasound systems in use today are of the _____ type.

5.8.14. Reflection-type instruments are also called _____ instruments.

5.8.15. Reflection-type instruments look for three things: the _____, _____, and arrival _____ of reflections that occur in tissues.

5.8.16. Doppler instruments look for the Doppler _____ of reflections that occur in tissues.

5.8.17. Imaging systems produce a visual _____ from the electrical _____ received from the transducer.

5.8.18. The transducer is connected to the display through the

_____.

5.8.19. The transducer receives voltages from the _____ in pulse-echo systems.

5.8.20. The _____ receives voltages from the transducer.

5.8.21. Increasing the gain generally produces the same effect as
a. decreasing the attenuation
b. increasing the attenuation
c. increasing the compression
d. increasing the rectification
e. both b and c

5.8.22. Voltage pulses occur at the output of the
    a. pulser
    b. transducer
    c. receiver
    d. display
    e. both a and b
    f. both c and e

5.8.23. Ultrasound pulses from the pulser are applied to the
    a. pulser
    b. transducer
    c. receiver
    d. display

5.8.24. Rectification and smoothing are parts of
    a. amplipression
    b. rejection
    c. a and b
    d. compression
    e. demodulation

5.8.25. If gain is reduced by one-half, and if input power is unchanged, the output power is _____ what it was before.
    a. equal to
    b. twice
    c. one-half
    d. none of the above

5.8.26. If gain was 30 dB and is reduced by one-half, the new gain is _____ dB.
    a. 15
    b. 60
    c. 33
    d. 27
    e. none of the above

5.8.27. If four shades of gray are shown on a display, each twice the brightness of the next brightest one, the brightest shade is _____ times the brightness of the dimmest shade.
    a. 2
    b. 4
    c. 8
    d. 16
    e. 32

5.8.28. The dynamic range displayed in Problem 5.8.27 is approximately _____ dB.
    a. 10   d. 2
    b. 9   e. 0
    c. 5

5.8.29. Gain and attenuation are usually given in
  a. dB
  b. dB/cm
  c. cm
  d. cm/3 dB
  e. none of the above

5.8.30. Compensation (swept gain) makes up for the fact that reflections from deeper reflectors arrive at the transducer with greater amplitude. True or false?

Chapter 6

Performance Measurements

6.1
Introduction

This chapter will describe devices and methods used to determine if diagnostic ultrasound imaging instruments are operating correctly and consistently. These devices and methods are considered in three groups: (1) those that test the operation of the instrument as a whole (imaging performance); (2) those that measure the acoustic output of the instrument; (3) those that measure the beam profiles produced by transducers. Group 1 takes into account the operations of all the components shown in Figure 5.2. Group 2 considers only the pulser and the transducer acting as a source. Group 3 considers only the transducer. In group 3 tests the transducer is driven and evaluated by a separate test generator or by the diagnostic instrument. Imaging performance is important for evaluating the instrument as a diagnostic tool. The acoustic output of an instrument is important when considering biological effects and safety (Chapter 7). Beam profiles are important when evaluating and choosing transducers.

6.2
Imaging
Performance

Imaging performance is determined by measuring the following parameters:
1. relative system **sensitivity**
2. longitudinal resolution (Section 3.7)
3. lateral resolution (Section 4.4)
4. **dead zone**
5. range (depth or distance) accuracy (Sections 3.6 and 5.4)

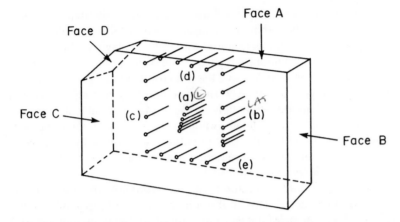

Figure 6.1. AIUM 100-mm test object. Rod groups are used for measuring (a) longitudinal resolution, (b) or (c) lateral resolution, (c) range accuracy and receiver compensation, (d) dead zone, and (a) through (e) registration accuracy. Any rod imaged may be used for sensitivity or dynamic range measurements.

6. **registration** accuracy
7. compensation (swept gain) operation (Section 5.3)
8. gray-scale dynamic range

These may all be measured using the 100-mm test object of the American Institute of Ultrasound in Medicine (AIUM) (Figure 6.1). This test object is composed of a series of 0.75-mm-diameter stainless-steel rods arranged in a pattern between two transparent plastic sides. The other sides are made of thin acrylic plastic sheets on which the transducer may be scanned using a coupling medium. The tank is filled with a mixture of alcohol, algae inhibitor, and water that has a propagation speed of 1.54 mm/μs at room temperature. The speed varies by less than 1 percent when temperature is changed by 5°C. Therefore, results with this test object are relatively insensitive to normal fluctuations in room temperature. Construction details and procedures for its use have been published.[10-12] These test objects are available commercially.

To obtain consistent measurements of longitudinal and lateral resolution and dead zone, even with a given transducer and diagnostic instrument, it is necessary to perform the test at consistent control settings. Usually it is best to measure relative system sensitivity first and then increase the sensitivity settings a fixed amount for performing the other tests.

Relative system sensitivity is a measure of how weak a reflection an instrument can display. It is obtained by finding the gain or attenuation setting (with no compensation) at which a particular rod in the test object produces a barely discernible display. Any imaged rod may be chosen for this measurement. Usually the top rod in group (a) or the bottom rod in group (c) is used for system sensitivity measurements (Figure 6.1). For the remaining measurements, 10 dB are added to the system sensitivity settings required to barely display the chosen rod.

Longitudinal resolution is measured with rod group (a). The transducer is placed on face A above the rod group. Not all the rods will be seen separately on the display. The spacing of the two closest rods in the group that are seen separately on the display is equal to the longitudinal resolution. Longitudinal resolution measured with the test object usually does not reflect the best possible resolution of the diagnostic system. However, the measurement is a consistency check for use with a given transducer and instrument.

Lateral resolution is measured with rod group (b). The transducer is scanned along face B. Not all the rods will be seen separately on the display. The spacing of the two closest rods in the group that are seen separately on the display is equal to the lateral resolution. Lateral resolution at ranges from 1 to 11 cm can be determined by measuring the width of the scan line for each rod in group (c) after the transducer is scanned across face A of the test object. If these measurements are to be used for more rigorous purposes than quality control, one must find the system sensitivity to display the rod of interest, increase the gain 6 dB, and then measure the lateral resolution by one of the methods previously described.

The dead zone is the distance closest to the transducer, in which imaging cannot be performed. It is measured with rod group (d). The transducer is scanned across face A. The distance from the transducer to the first rod imaged is equal to the dead zone.

Range accuracy is measured with rod group (c). The rods should appear on the display at 1, 3, 5, 7, 9, and 11 cm from the transducer. Relative distances between the rods should be accurate to at least 2 mm. The space between the rods at 1 and 11 cm should be recorded with calipers and then measured with marker dots placed parallel to rod group (e). If this indicates that the distance between the rods at 1 and 11 cm differs from the true 10 cm by more than 2 mm, then the horizontal and vertical display scales are not identical. In that case, marker dots are placed exactly at the location and orientation of any critical distance measurement, such as that of biparietal diameter.

Registration is the positioning of reflectors on the display. It depends on transmission of proper transducer location and orientation information, using the dash path in Figure 5.2, and on satisfactory range accuracy, as described previously. Registration accuracy is measured using all the rods and scanning over faces A, B, C, and D. Correct registration results in star-shaped images at the location of each rod. Registration error is measured as the greatest separation between centers of any two lines in the image of any rod.[11]

Compensation operation is measured using rod group (c). The transducer is placed on face A above this rod group. With no compensation, the attenuator or gain settings required to display each rod at a given pulse height (A mode) or gray level (B, C, or M mode) are recorded. This is then done again with compensation on. The difference between the settings for each rod as a function of distance is the compensation characteristic.

The gray-scale dynamic range is the difference between gain or attenuator settings (dB) that produce (1) barely discernible and (2) maximum deflection (A mode) or brightness (B, C, or M mode) displays for the same reflection. Any rod imaged may be chosen for this measurement.

6.2.1. The 100-mm test object contains several stainless-steel *.75M stain Rods* immersed in a mixture of algae inhibitor, *Alcohol*____, and *water*_____ that has a propagation speed 1.54 mm/μs.

6.2.2. Match the parameters measured with the rod groups used (Figure 6.1) (answers may be used more than once):
   a. longitudinal resolution: *1*
   b. lateral resolution: *2*
   c. range accuracy: *3*
   d. registration accuracy: *6*
   e. dead zone: *4*
   f. compensation: *3*
   g. sensitivity: _____
   h. dynamic range: *7*

   1. rod group (a)
   2. rod group (b)
   3. rod group (c)
   4. rod group (d)
   5. rod group (e)
   6. all rods
   7. any rod

6.2.3. Match the parameters measured with the types of observation modes (answers may be used more than once):
   a. longitudinal resolution: _____
   b. lateral resolution: _____
   c. range accuracy: _____
   d. registration accuracy: _____
   e. dead zone: _____
   f. compensation: _____
   g. sensitivity: _____
   h. dynamic range: _____

   1. gain or attenuator settings
   2. first rod imaged
   3. star-shaped images
   4. rod distances from transducer in the display
   5. minimum spacing of separately displayed rods

6.2.4. Test objects are available commercially. True or false?

6.2.5. Results using a test object are relatively insensitive to temperature. True or false?

6.2.6. The speed of sound in the recommended alcohol and water mixture of the AIUM test object varies by less than *1.0* percent when the temperature is changed by 5°C.

6.3
Acoustic
Output

Several devices or phenomena are used for measuring the acoustic output of diagnostic instruments. They are listed in Table 6.1 with the parameters they are used to measure.

The **hydrophone** (also called a microprobe) is a small (1-mm diameter or less) transducer element mounted on the end of a narrow tube or hollow needle (Figure 6.2). Its size causes it to receive sound reasonably well from all directions without altering the sound by its presence. In response to the varying pressure of the sound, it produces a varying voltage that can be displayed on an oscilloscope. A picture similar to that in Figure 2.7 is produced, from which period, pulse repetition period, and pulse duration can be determined. From these quantities, frequency, pulse repetition frequency, and duty factor can be calculated. If the hydrophone calibration is known (relationship between voltage produced and pressure applied), pressure amplitude may also be determined. If propagation speed is known, wavelength and spatial pulse length can be calculated (Sections 2.2 and 2.3). If impedance is known, intensity can be calculated. Probe calibration factors have not been adequate in the past to make highly accurate determination of pressure and intensity, but there is promise that this situation will improve. Hydrophones are commercially available and are relatively inexpensive and simple to use.

Acousto-optics concerns the interaction between light and sound. Density variations in a sound wave can refract light. By properly receiving the refracted light, a picture similar to that in Figure 2.7 can be displayed on an oscilloscope. From this, the density amplitude, period, pulse repetition period, and pulse duration may be measured. From these quantities, frequency, pulse repetition frequency, duty factor, wavelength, spatial pulse length, and intensity may be calculated. A second system, the **schlieren** (German for shadow) system, uses acousto-optic interaction to display a two-dimensional cross section of

Table 6.1

Devices and Phenomena Used to Measure
Acoustic Output Parameters

Device or phenomenon	Parameters measured
Hydrophone	amplitude
	period
	pulse duration
	pulse repetition period
Acousto-optics	amplitude
	period
	pulse duration
	pulse repetition period
Radiation force	power or intensity
Calorimeter	energy
Thermocouple	intensity

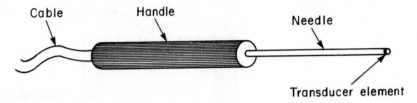

Figure 6.2. A hydrophone consists of a small transducer element mounted on the end of a needle.

the beam shape produced by an ultrasound transducer. This cross section is along the direction of propagation. Acousto-optic systems are not commercially available and are not simple to use.

Radiation force is exerted on an absorbing or reflecting object on which a sound beam is incident. The force is proportional to the power in the sound beam. Three devices are used for measuring radiation force (Figure 6.3):

1. balance
2. float
3. suspended ball

For pulsed ultrasound, the first two devices respond to time-averaged power. If beam area is known, spatial average intensity can be calculated from acoustic power (Section 2.4). For pulsed ultrasound, the calculated intensity is the SATA value. The third device yields the intensity at its location in the beam. By properly locating the ball in the beam, the SPTA intensity may be measured. Radiation force devices are commercially available and are relatively inexpensive and simple to use.

A **calorimeter** measures the temperature rise in an absorbing liquid (Figure 6.4). From this, the total energy absorbed by the liquid can be calculated. Power can be calculated if exposure time is known (Ap-

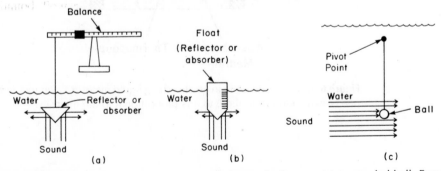

Figure 6.3. Radiation force is measured by (a) balance, (b) float, or (c) suspended ball. Force is measured (a) by the balance reading, (b) by the amount the float is pushed out of the water, or (c) by the amount the ball is pushed to the side.

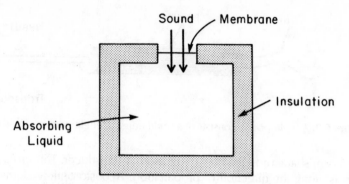

Figure 6.4. A calorimeter absorbs all the energy of a sound beam. The temperature rise of the absorbing liquid is proportional to the total energy absorbed.

pendix 2). Then intensity can be calculated if beam area is known (Section 2.4). Calorimeters are not commercially available and are not simple to use.

A small **thermocouple** embedded in an absorbing medium (Figure 6.5) can be used to measure intensity at a point. The intensity is proportional to the rate of temperature rise measured by the thermocouple when the sound is turned on. Thermocouples are less sensitive than hydrophones. Thermocouple measurement systems are not commercially available and are not simple to use.

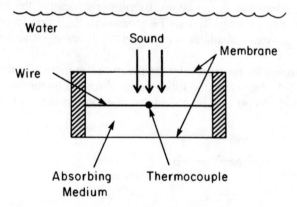

Figure 6.5. A thermocouple in an absorbing liquid measures a temperature rise rate (when sound is applied) that is proportional to the intensity.

6.3.1. Match the following devices or phenomena with the parameters measured (answers may be used more than once):
    a. hydrophone: _____,
    _____, _____, _____
    b. acousto-optics: _____,
    _____, _____, _____
    c. radiation force: _____,
    _____
    d. calorimeter: _____
    e. thermocouple: _____

    1. power
    2. intensity
    3. energy
    4. amplitude
    5. period
    6. pulse duration
    7. pulse repetition period

6.3.2. Match the following (answers may be used more than once):
    a. hydrophone: _____
    b. acousto-optics: _____
    c. radiation force: _____
    d. calorimeter: _____
    e. thermocouple: _____

    1. commercially available
    2. not simple to use

6.3.3. A hydrophone contains a small ___Transducer___ element.

6.3.4. Because of small size, the following can measure spatial details of a sound beam:
    a. hydrophone ✓
    b. calorimeter
    c. thermocouple
    d. both a and b
    e. both a and c

6.3.5. Match the following:
    a. hydrophone: _____
    b. acousto-optics: _____
    c. radiation force: _____
    d. calorimeter: _____
    e. thermocouple: _____

    1. interaction with light
    2. produces a voltage
    3. measures intensity
    4. measured with balance, float, or ball
    5. measures total energy

6.3.6. Match the following (A can be calculated from B if C is known) (answers may be used more than once):

A:

a. frequency: _____, _____, _____
b. pulse repetition frequency: _____, _____
c. duty factor: _____, _____
d. wavelength: _____, _____
e. spatial pulse length: _____, _____
f. power: _____, _____
g. intensity: _____, _____

B:
1. wavelength
2. period
3. pulse repetition period
4. frequency
5. energy
6. power

C:
7. number of cycles in the pulse
8. pulse duration
9. propagation speed
10. exposure time
11. beam area
12. nothing else

**6.4
Beam
Profile**

The test object described in Section 6.2 measures one beam parameter, the beam diameter, which is equal to lateral resolution. However, it does this only at one distance from the transducer: the distance from face B to rod group (b) in Figure 6.1. The use of rod group (c) in Figure 6.1 does not suffer from this same restriction. However, there is some distortion of the lateral resolution measurements in rod group (c) because of shadowing of lower rods by rods in the focal region. The test object is used to make this measurement using the ultrasound imaging instrument as a whole (the rod reflections are imaged on the instrument display). A **beam profiler** is a device designed to give three-dimensional reflection amplitude information. It uses a set of rods at various distances from the transducer (Figure 6.6). The transducer is pulsed as it is scanned across the tank. Reflections are received from each rod, and voltage amplitude is measured. As the sound beam passes over a rod, the reflected amplitude increases, goes through a maximum, and then decreases. Then the next rod (at a greater distance) is encountered, with a similar reflection behavior. This continues until all rods have been encountered. A beam profile can be plotted from this procedure (Figure 6.7). A beam profile does not actually give a profile of a beam, i.e., it does not plot acoustic amplitude or intensity across the beam at several distances from the transducer as it appears to do. It actually plots reflection amplitude received at the

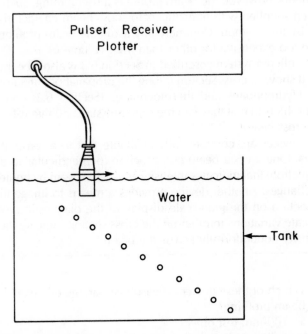

Figure 6.6. A beam profiler consists of a pulser, receiver, plotter, transducer, and tank with rods at various distances from the transducer. The transducer is scanned over the rods.

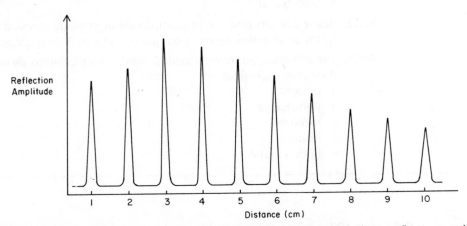

Figure 6.7. Beam profile plotted by the system in Figure 6.6. Each peak shows reflection amplitude as scanned across the rod that is at the distance indicated from the transducer. The amplitude is maximum at the near-zone length of an unfocused transducer (Section 4.3) or the focal region of a focused transducer (Section 4.4).

transducer, and it could be called a reflection profiler. For imaging instruments, however, the beam profile is a useful thing. Such profiles are often supplied with transducers to show beam characteristics obtained by this method. Commercially available beam profilers generally are too expensive for other than high-volume users.

The schlieren system described in Section 6.3 is also a beam profiler in that it shows a cross section (along the propagation direction) of the beam. Hydrophones and thermocouples (Section 6.3) can also be beam profilers in that they can measure pressure and intensity distributions across beams.

Two devices are commercially available that in a sense are beam profilers. One gives a beam cross section (perpendicular to propagation direction) that indicates intensity across the beam by liquid-crystal color changes. Another device provides a means to image the beam cross section on the gray-scale display of the diagnostic instrument. Gray-scale variations throughout the cross section indicate the degree of intensity nonuniformity across the beam.

Exercises

6.4.1. Which of these devices measure(s) parameters related to beam profiling?
a. 100-mm test object
b. radiation force balance
c. schlieren system
d. both a and c
e. both b and c

6.4.2. Beam profilers plot acoustic amplitude or intensity across the beam at several distances from the transducer. True or false?

6.4.3. The following are often supplied with beam profiles to show their characteristics:
a. pulsers
b. transducers
c. receivers
d. displays
e. both a and c

6.5 Review The 100-mm test object provides a means of measuring longitudinal and lateral resolution, range and registration accuracy, dead zone, compensation, sensitivity, and dynamic range of diagnostic instruments. Hydrophones, acousto-optics, radiation force, calorimeters, and thermocouples are used to measure the acoustic output of diagnostic instruments. Beam profilers measure characteristics of beams produced by transducers.

6.5.1. Match these devices or phenomena with what they measure (answers may be used more than once):

a. beam profiler: _____
b. 100-mm test object:

_____, _____

c. hydrophone: _____,

_____

d. balance or float: _____
e. calorimeter: _____
f. thermocouple: _____,

_____

1. diagnostic instrument imaging performance
2. transducer beam characteristics
3. diagnostic instrument acoustic output

6.5.2. Match the following with the components they usually provide information about:

a. radiation force and calorimetry: _____
b. beam profiler: _____
c. 100-mm test object:

_____

1. diagnostic instrument as a whole
2. pulser and transducer
3. transducer
4. transducer and receiver
5. receiver and display

Chapter 7

Bioeffects and Safety

7.1
Introduction

The interaction between ultrasound and tissues is pictured in Figure 1.1. The aspect of the acoustic propagation properties of the interaction was discussed in Chapters 2 and 3. The aspect of the biological effects will be discussed in this chapter. This aspect is useful in therapy applications of ultrasound. We shall not consider this subject here. Of concern to us in diagnostic ultrasound is what the biological effects of ultrasound tell us about the safety or hazard of the diagnostic ultrasound method. What we would like to do is ask the question "Is it safe?" and give the answer "Yes." If this were possible, a separate chapter on the subject would not be needed. This ideal situation is not necessary for the procedure to be useful. We do not apply such a strong criterion to other areas of life. We cannot say that riding in a car is safe; yet we choose to go off in one daily. What we desire is knowledge of the probability of damage or injury and under what conditions this probability is maximized (in order to avoid those conditions) and minimized (in order to seek those conditions). In any diagnostic test there may be some risk (some probability of damage or injury). For diagnostic ultrasound, the physician and sonographer need to know something about this risk. Risk can be weighed against benefit in determining the appropriateness of the diagnostic procedure in each case. Knowledge of how to minimize the risk is useful to everyone involved in diagnostic ultrasound.

We do not know what we would like to know: What types of injury can diagnostic ultrasound produce in patients? Under what conditions? Sufficient epidemiologic data are not available.[13,14]

What we do know is something about biological effects in experimental animals. Hundreds of reports on this subject have appeared in the scientific literature. Some reviews of this subject are contained herein.[2,4,15-19] Attempts have been made to define hazardous and nonhazardous conditions based on these data.[16,17]

The Biological Effects Committee of the American Institute of Ultrasound in Medicine (AIUM) has reviewed the reports of biological effects of ultrasound and formulated the following statement:[20]

Statement on Mammalian In Vivo Ultrasonic Biological Effects
October 1978
In the low megahertz frequency range there have been no independently confirmed significant biological effects in mammalian tissues exposed to intensities* below 100 mW/cm². Furthermore, for ultrasonic exposure times** less than 500 seconds and greater than one second, such effects have not been demonstrated even at higher intensities, when the product of intensity* and exposure time** is less than 50 joules/cm².

*Spatial peak, temporal average as measured in a free field in water.
**Total time; this includes off-time as well as on-time for a repeated-pulse regime.

The low-megahertz range referred to in this statement is 0.5–10 MHz. The intensity considered is the SPTA intensity discussed in Section 2.4. "Measured in a free field" means that there were no reflections from the walls of the measuring system. "Repeated-pulse regime" (pulsed ultrasound) is discussed in Section 2.3. The product of intensity and time is:

intensity × time

$$= \left[\frac{\text{power}}{\text{beam area}} \right] \times \left[\text{time} \right] \qquad \text{(Section 2.4)}$$

$$= \left[\frac{\text{energy}}{\text{time}} \right] \times \left[\frac{\text{time}}{\text{beam area}} \right] \qquad \text{(Appendix 2)}$$

$$= \frac{\text{energy}}{\text{beam area}} \quad (\text{J/cm}^2) \qquad \text{(Table A5.1)}$$

This is the energy passed through an area divided by the area.

This statement describes intensity and time limits below which "independently confirmed significant" biological effects have not been reported. These limits are shown in Figure 7.1. They are probably not minimum or threshold levels. As more sensitive biological end points are studied, it is reasonable to expect some lowering of these levels.

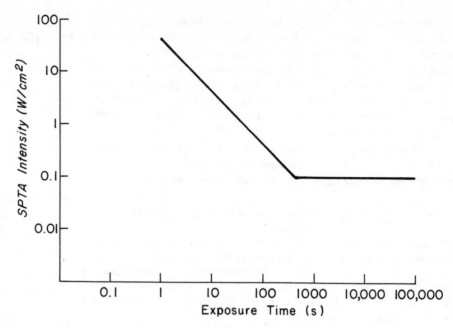

Figure 7.1. Intensity and time limits described by the AIUM statement on mammalian in vivo ultrasound biological effects. There are no independently confirmed significant biological effects in mammalian tissues for intensity and time conditions below the line. Intensity is SPTA as measured in a free field in water. Time is total time of exposure to ultrasound (includes time between pulses in the case of pulsed ultrasound).

Reports used in determining the preceding statement considered the following biological effects (see Section 5.2 of Nyborg[19]): hind-limb paralysis, fetal weight reduction, postpartum mortality, and liver mitotic index reduction, all in mice and rats; blood vessel damage in chick embryos; wound healing in rabbit ears; postulated human fetal abnormalities based on absorption heating. The results were obtained with focused beams as well as unfocused beams, generated continuously or (to a lesser extent) as pulsed ultrasound.

A comparison of the instrument output data from Table 5.2 with the bioeffects statement levels is given in Figure 7.2. In making this comparison, the pulsed ultrasound of the instruments is compared with the continuous sound used in most bioeffects studies. This is done by using the SPTA intensity of the pulsed ultrasound. If bioeffects depend on temporal average intensity, this is a valid comparison.

Three mechanisms of action for ultrasound bioeffects are generally recognized:

1. heat
2. **cavitation**
3. other

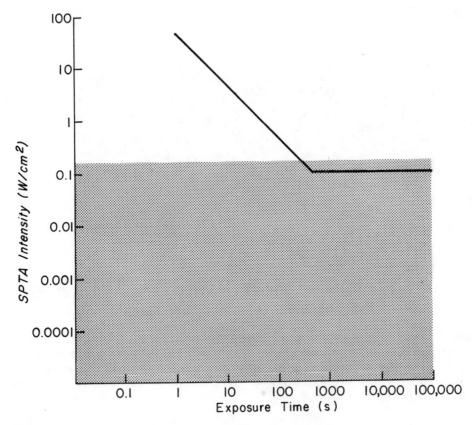

Figure 7.2. Comparison of instrument output data with AIUM bioeffects statement level. The shaded area shows the range in which diagnostic instruments fall (Table 5.2). SPTA intensity is used, assuming that temporal average is relevant. Time is total time of exposure to ultrasound (includes time between pulses in the case of pulsed ultrasound).

The third class is sometimes called mechanical. Little is known about it. For our purpose, it really means nonthermal and noncavitational. Heating depends on temporal average intensity. Cavitation does not. The intensity dependence of the category "other" is unknown.

The overlap in Figure 7.2 suggests that with the instruments that operate at the higher intensities it may be possible to produce some biological effects in small animals.

Another means of comparison is shown in Figure 7.3, where the SPTP intensity range of Table 5.2 is used. This assumes that individual pulses (typically 2–6 cycles long) can produce a bioeffect, that they add up (repair or recovery between pulses does not occur), and thus that bioeffects depend on temporal peak intensity. Whether or not any of this is true under any conditions is not currently known. If it were true, the overlap in Figure 7.3 would indicate that times greater than

135

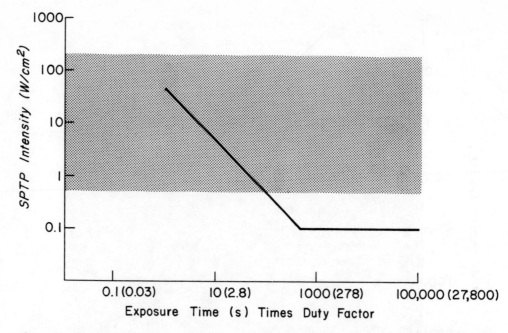

Figure 7.3. Comparison of instrument data with AIUM bioeffects statement level. SPTP intensity is used (for pulsed ultrasound), assuming that temporal peak is relevant. The shaded area shows the range in which diagnostic instruments fall (Table 5.2). Time is sound-on time (total exposure time multiplied by duty factor for pulsed ultrasound). Exposure time in hours (assuming that the duty factor is 0.001) is given in parentheses.

1–50 s (depending on the SPTP intensity of the instrument) could produce biological effects in animals. In this case the appropriate time is the sound-on time, which is total exposure time multiplied by duty factor (typically 0.001–0.003). Total exposure times corresponding to 1–50 s sound-on time are (assuming a duty factor of 0.001) 1000–50,000 s (17 min to 14 hr).

Another consideration in these comparisons is whether or not sound exposures separated by several hours or days add up (repair or recovery does not occur between exposures). No data are available to permit any statement on this consideration.

7.3 Safety

For consideration of the safety of diagnostic ultrasound, we must try to relate our bioeffects knowledge to the clinical situation. There are three questions that arise when we attempt to accomplish this:

1. Do any of the bioeffects that have occurred under experimental conditions constitute a hazard to a human in the clinical setting?

2. Are the acoustic parameters at the site of the bioeffect in experimental animals comparable to those at the appropriate site of concern in the body during diagnosis?
3. Do the continuous-wave conditions of most experimental studies provide any useful information for the pulsed ultrasound of clinical diagnosis?

These questions remain largely unanswered. Being unable to give a satisfying response to question 1, we must attempt to determine if *any* bioeffects observed in experimental animals are likely to occur clinically. This brings us to the difficulties of questions 2 and 3. The response to question 2 is that in human applications of ultrasound, the organs of concern are normally farther from the sound source (a longer attenuating sound path is involved). Also, a smaller organ volume fraction is exposed because the organs are larger than those of the experimental animals. Experimental studies are normally done with a stationary sound beam, whereas diagnostic studies usually involve scanning. These considerations may provide some (unknown) safety factors for the diagnostic situation. Question 3 was considered in the discussion of Figure 7.3.

Not knowing all the things we would like to know, we must take a conservative approach to safety considerations: *Use diagnostic ultrasound in an appropriate manner when benefit is expected from the procedure.* This is easier said than done. Listed here are four items of advice included in the AIUM brochure[21] on the subject:

1. Look for output intensity specifications when considering equipment for purchase.
2. If two instruments seem comparable in other respects, choose the one with the lowest intensity.
3. Balance benefit against risk. The AIUM statement does not indicate that SPTA intensity greater than 100 mW/cm² should never be used or that lower values are "safe." If a higher intensity can provide necessary information, it should be used. Use diagnostic ultrasound only when benefit is expected. Use the minimum exposure (intensity and time) to achieve the benefit.
4. One should not be hesitant to use ultrasound, with appropriate equipment and procedures, when benefit is expected. Diagnostic ultrasound has proved itself to be an effective tool in medical practice. We can take considerable satisfaction in the fact that after years of accumulated experience in the clinical use of diagnostic ultrasound there has been no known instance of human injury caused by it. This is, indeed, an excellent safety record. By thoughtful and judicious use of the technique, we can help to maintain this record.

7.4
Review

The AIUM has stated that there have been no independently confirmed significant biological effects in mammalian tissues exposed to SPTA intensities below 100 mW/cm². This indicates that with some instruments that operate at the higher intensities, it may be possible to produce some biological effects in small animals. Whether or not they can occur in humans is unknown. Not knowing what we need to know to be more specific, we take the conservative approach: Use diagnostic ultrasound in an appropriate manner when benefit is expected from the procedure.

Exercises

7.4.1. There is no possible hazard involved in the diagnostic use of ultrasound. True or false?

7.4.2. Ultrasound should not be used as a diagnostic tool because of the bioeffects it can produce. True or false?

7.4.3. No independently confirmed significant biological effects in mammalian tissues have been reported at intensities below
a. 10 W/cm² SPTP
b. 100 mW/cm² SPTA
c. 10 mW/cm² SPTA
d. 10 mW/cm² SATA
e. 1 mW/cm² SATP

7.4.4. Do we know what types of injuries ultrasound might produce in patients, and under what conditions? NO

7.4.5. Do we know of any biological effects that ultrasound can produce in small animals under experimental conditions? yes

7.4.6. Heating depends on
a. SATA intensity
b. SATP intensity
c. SPTP intensity

7.4.7. When SPTA intensities of pulsed and continuous-wave ultrasound are compared, the appropriate time to be used is
a. the total exposure time
b. the sound-on time

7.4.8. When SPTP intensity of pulsed ultrasound is compared with SPTA intensity of continuous-wave ultrasound, the appropriate time to be used is
a. the total exposure time
b. the sound-on time

138

7.4.9. The sound-on time is the total time multiplied by
   a. SP/SA ratio
   b. pulse repetition frequency
   c. Doppler shift
   d. reflection coefficient
   e. duty factor

7.4.10. The available epidemiologic data are sufficient to make a final judgment on the safety of diagnostic ultrasound. True or false?

Chapter 8

Summary

By sending short pulses of ultrasound into the body and using reflections received from tissue interfaces to produce images of internal structures, ultrasound is used as a medical diagnostic tool. Ultrasound is a wave of traveling acoustic variables described by frequency, period, wavelength, propagation speed, amplitude, intensity, and attenuation. Pulsed ultrasound is used in ultrasound imaging. It is described, additionally, by pulse repetition frequency and period, duty factor, and spatial pulse length. Diagnostic ultrasound commonly uses frequencies from 1 to 10 MHz, SPTA intensities from 0.01 to 200 mW/cm², pulse repetition frequencies of approximately 1 kHz, duty factors from 0.001 to 0.003, and pulses of from 2 to 6 cycles. Soft-tissue propagation speed is 1.54 mm/μs, and the attenuation coefficient is 1 dB/cm for each megahertz of frequency. For *normal incidence* at boundaries, reflections are produced if media impedances (density times propagation speed) are different. For *oblique incidence,* refraction occurs if media propagation speeds are different. For *oblique incidence,* reflections depend on media propagation speeds and densities. A Doppler shift is produced if the boundary is moving. The distance to reflectors is determined by round-trip travel time. Reverberations are generated between reflectors.

Transducers convert electrical energy to ultrasound energy and vice versa by piezoelectricity. Longitudinal resolution (acoustic) is equal to one-half the spatial pulse length, which can be reduced by damping.

Lateral resolution (acoustic) is equal to beam diameter, which can be reduced by focusing. These resolutions (with focusing) are approximately 1 mm. Imaging system resolutions are usually worse than this. Disc transducers produce sound beams with near and far zones. Arrays can scan, steer, and shape beams repeatedly, permitting real-time imaging. Real-time imaging can also be accomplished with mechanically driven single-element transducers.

Pulse-echo systems use the amplitude, direction, and arrival time of reflections to produce A, B, C, or M mode displays. Imaging systems consist of pulser, transducer, receiver, and display. Pulsers set the pulse repetition frequency, which determines maximum imaging depth. Scan converters store gray-scale image information and permit display on a television monitor. Reverberation, shadowing, enhancement, curved or oblique reflectors, propagation speed error, refraction, side lobes, multipath, and the resolution produce display artifacts. Doppler systems use the Doppler shift of reflections to produce audible sound, characteristic of motion.

Imaging performance is measured with the AIUM 100-mm test object. Acoustic output is measured with hydrophone, acousto-optics, radiation force, calorimetry, and thermocouple. Beam profilers, test objects, hydrophones, thermocouples, and schlieren systems measure transducer beam characteristics.

There have been no independently confirmed significant biological effects in mammalian tissues exposed to SPTA intensities below 100 mW/cm^2. Diagnostic ultrasound should be used in an appropriate manner when benefit is to be expected from the information gained.

Exercises

8.1. Increasing the frequency
   a. improves resolution
   b. increases the depth of penetration
   c. increases refraction
   d. both a and b
   e. both a and c

8.2. Increasing the pulse repetition frequency
   a. improves resolution
   b. increases maximum depth imaged
   c. decreases maximum depth imaged
   d. both a and b
   e. both a and c

8.3. Increasing the intensity produced by the transducer
    a. is accomplished by increasing the pulser voltage
    b. increases the sensitivity of the system
    c. increases the probability of biological effects
  ✓d. all of the above
    e. none of the above

8.4. Increasing the spatial pulse length
    a. is accomplished by transducer damping
    b. is accompanied by decreased pulse duration
    c. improves longitudinal resolution
    d. all of the above
    e. none of the above

8.5. Real-time imaging is made possible by
    a. scan converters
  ✓b. mechanically driven transducers
    c. gray-scale display
    d. arrays
    e. both b and d

8.6. The 100-mm test object measures
  ✓a. resolution
    b. pulse duration
    c. SATA intensity
    d. wavelength
    e. all of the above

8.7. The following measure acoustic power:
    a. hydrophone
    b. acousto-optics
    c. 100-mm test object
    d. all of the above
    e. none of the above

8.8. Ultrasound bioeffects
    a. do not occur
    b. do not occur with diagnostic instruments
  ✓c. are not confirmed below 100 mW/cm^2 SPTA
    d. both b and c
    e. none of the above

8.9. The diagnostic ultrasound frequency range is
    a. 1–10 mHz
    b. 1–10 kHz
  ✓c. 1–10 MHz
    d. 3–15 kHz
    e. none of the above

8.10. Small transducers always produce smaller beam diameters. True or false?

8.11. No reflection occurs if media impedances are equal. True or false?

8.12. No refraction occurs if media impedances are equal. True or false?

8.13. Gray-scale display is made possible by
    a. array transducers
    b. cathode-ray storage tubes
    ✓c. scan converters
    d. both b and c
    e. all of the above

8.14. Attenuation is corrected for by
    a. demodulation
    b. desegregation
    c. decompression
    ✓d. compensation
    e. remuneration

8.15. Vertical deflections of the display spot are produced by reflections in
    a. the B mode
    b. the C mode
    c. the M mode
    d. the à la mode
    ✓e. none of the above

8.16. This textbook is
    a. enjoyable
    b. profitable
    c. relevant
    d. well done
    e. complete
    f. accurate
    g. concise
    h. stimulating
    i. simple
    j. clear
    k. error-freee
    m. omission-free
    o. helpful
    p. perfect
    q. great
    r. all of the above

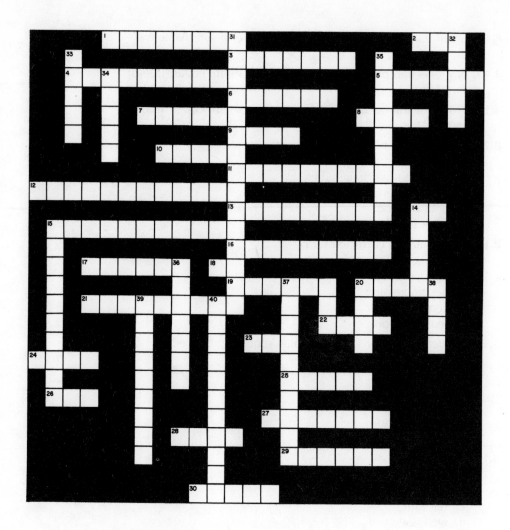

8.17 Across:
1. Referring to sound
2. Abbreviation for cosine
3. Not perpendicular to a boundary
4. Occurs at boundaries with normal incidence
5. Material through which sound is passing
6. The C mode requires _____ the receiver
7. The duty _____ is sound-on fraction
8. Beam diameter decreases in the _____ zone
9. Intensity is power divided by beam _____
10. Reflector motion produces a Doppler _____
11. Sound of frequency 20 kHz and higher
12. Parallel to sound direction

13. Maximum variation of an acoustic variable
14. Abbreviation for continuous wave
15. Attenuation _____ is given decibels per centimeter
16. Power divided by beam area
17. Reciprocal of frequency
18. The range equation gives distance _____ a reflector
19. Perpendicular to a boundary
20. Displacement divided by time
21. Propagation speed depends on density and _____
22. _____ scale displays several values of spot brightness
23. Beam diameter increases in the _____ zone
24. Force times displacement
25. Longitudinal resolution depends on spatial _____ length
26. Abbreviation for sine
27. Reflected frequency minus incident frequency equals _____ shift
28. A traveling variation
29. Capabililty of doing work
30. Complete variation of a wave variable

Down:

14. One hertz is one _____ per second
15. The abbreviation cw stands for _____ wave
20. A line produced on a display is called a _____ line
31. (A message for you)
32. Traveling wave of acoustic variables
33. Transducer assembly containing more than one element
34. _____ length is the distance from a focused transducer to minimum beam diameter
35. Density times propagation speed
36. Mass divided by volume
37. Another name for a hydrophone
38. Pulse duration divided by burst repetition period is _____ factor
39. Reciprocal of period
40. Ability of an imaging system to detect weak reflections

Glossary

The terms defined here are printed in boldface at first appearance in this textbook. The American National Standards Institute[22] has provided definitions more rigorous than the simplified ones given here.

Absorption. Conversion of sound to heat.

Acceleration. Change in velocity divided by time over which the change occurs.

Acoustics. Having to do with sound.

Acoustic propagation properties. Characteristics of a medium that affect the propagation of sound through it.

Acoustic variables. Pressure, density, temperature, and particle motion—things that are functions of space and time in a sound wave.

Acousto-optics. Interaction of light and sound.

A mode. Mode of operation in which the display records a vertical spot deflection for each pulse delivered from the receiver.

Amplification. Increasing small voltages to larger ones.

Amplifier. A device that accomplishes amplification.

Amplitude. Maximum variation of an acoustic variable or voltage.

Annular array. Array made up of ring-shaped elements arranged concentrically.

Attenuation. Decrease in amplitude and intensity as a wave travels through a medium.

Attenuation coefficient. Attenuation per unit length of wave travel.

Array. Transducer array.

Backscatter. Sound scattered back in the direction from which it originally came.

Bandwidth. Range of frequencies involved in an ultrasound pulse.

Beam area. Cross-sectional area of a sound beam.

Beam profiler. A device that plots three-dimensional reflection amplitude information.

Bistable display. Display in which all recorded spots have the same brightness.

B mode. Mode of operation in which the display records a spot brightening for each pulse delivered from the receiver, producing a cross-sectional image through the scanning plane (B scan).

B scan. An image that is a cross section of the object through the scanning plane.

Calorimeter. A device that measures temperature rise due to energy absorbed in a liquid.

Cathode-ray tube. A display device that produces an image by scanning an electron beam over a phosphor-coated screen.

Cavitation (acoustic). Production and behavior of bubbles in sound.

Compensation. Equalizing received reflection amplitude differences due to reflector depth.

C mode. Mode of operation in which the display records a spot brightening for each pulse delivered from the receiver, producing a cross-sectional image parallel to the body surface (C scan).

Compression. Decreasing differences between small and large amplitudes.

Continuous mode. Continuous-wave mode.

Continuous wave. A wave in which cycles repeat indefinitely, not pulsed.

Continuous-wave mode. Mode of operation in which continuous-wave sound is used.

cos. Abbreviation for cosine.

Cosine. The cosine of angle A in Figure A3.1 is the length of side b divided by the length of side c.

Coupling medium. Oil or gel used to provide a good sound path between the transducer and the skin.

C scan. An image that is a cross section of the object parallel to the surface and at a depth selected by gating.

cw. Abbreviation for continuous wave.

Cycle. Complete variation of an acoustic variable.

Damping. Material placed behind the rear face of a transducer element to reduce pulse duration; also, the process of pulse duration reduction.

dB. Abbreviation for decibel.

Dead zone. Distance closest to the transducer in which imaging cannot be performed.

Decibel. Unit of power or intensity ratio; the number of decibels is 10 times the logarithm (to the base 10) of the power or intensity ratio.

Demodulation. Converting voltage pulses from one form to another.

Density. Mass divided by volume.

Depth of penetration. Depth in tissue at which intensity is reduced to some fraction (e.g., one-half) of what it was at the surface.

Disc. Thin flat circular object.

Displacement. Distance that an object has moved.

Doppler effect. Frequency change of reflected sound wave due to reflector motion relative to transducer.

Doppler shift. Reflected frequency minus incident frequency.

Duty factor. Fraction of time that pulsed ultrasound is actually on.

Dynamic range. Ratio (in dB) of largest power to smallest power that a system can handle.

Echo. Reflection.

Effective reflecting area. The area of a reflector from which sound is received by a transducer.

Electrical pulse. A brief excursion of electrical voltage from its normal value.

Energy. Capability of doing work.

Enhancement. Increase in reflection amplitude from reflectors that lie behind a weakly attenuating structure.

Far zone. The region of a sound beam in which the beam diameter increases as the distance from the transducer increases.

Focal length. Distance from focused transducer to center of focal region or to the location of the spatial peak intensity.

Focal region. Region of minimum beam diameter and area.

Focus. To concentrate the sound beam into a smaller beam area than would exist without focusing.

Force. That which changes the state of rest or motion of an object.

Frame. Display image produced by one complete scan of the sound beam.

Frame rate. Number of frames displayed per unit time.

Frequency. Number of cycles per unit time.

Gain. Ratio of output to input electrical power.

Gating (pulsed Doppler). Passing only short pulses of voltage to the transducer from the voltage generator.

Gating (receiver). Passing only reflections that arrive at a certain time after the transducer produces a pulse.

Gray-scale display. Display in which several values of spot brightness may be displayed.

Heat. Energy due to thermal molecular motion.

Hertz. Unit of frequency, one cycle per second; unit of pulse repetition frequency, one pulse per second.

Hydrophone. A small transducer element mounted on the end of a narrow tube.

Hz. Abbreviation for hertz.

Incidence angle. Angle between incident sound direction and line perpendicular to media boundary.

Impedance. Density multiplied by sound propagation speed.

Intensity. Power divided by beam area.

Intensity reflection coefficient. Reflected intensity divided by incident intensity.

Intensity transmission coefficient. Transmitted intensity divided by incident intensity.

kHz. Abbreviation for kilohertz.

Kilohertz. One thousand hertz.

Lateral. Perpendicular to the direction of sound travel.

Lateral resolution. Minimum reflector separation perpendicular to the sound path required for separate reflections to be produced.

Linear array. Array made up of rectangular elements in a line.

Linear phased array. Linear array operated by applying voltage pulses to all elements, but with small time differences.

Linear switched array. Linear array operated by applying voltage pulses to groups of elements sequentially.

log. Abbreviation for logarithm.

Logarithm. The logarithm of a number is equal to 1 plus the number of times 10 must be multiplied by itself to result in that number.

Longitudinal. Along the direction of sound travel.

Longitudinal resolution. Minimum reflector separation along the sound path required for separate reflections to be produced.

Longitudinal wave. Wave in which the particle motion is parallel to the direction of wave travel.

Mass. Measure of an object's resistance to acceleration.

Matching layer. Material placed in front of the front face of a transducer element to reduce the reflection at the transducer surface.

Medium. Material through which a wave travels.

Megahertz. One million hertz.

MHz. Abbreviation for megahertz.

M mode. Mode of operation in which the display records a spot brightening for each pulse delivered from the receiver, producing a one-dimensional time display of reflector position (motion).

Multipath. Paths to and from a reflector are not the same.

Multiple reflection. Several reflections produced by a pulse encountering a pair of reflectors.

Near zone. The region of a sound beam in which the beam diameter decreases as the distance from the transducer increases.

Normal incidence. Sound direction is perpendicular to media boundary.

Oblique incidence. Sound direction is not perpendicular to media boundary.

Operating frequency. Preferred frequency of operation of a transducer.

Particle. Small portion of a medium.

Particle motion. Displacement, speed, velocity, and acceleration of a particle.

Period. Time per cycle.

Piezoelectricity. Conversion of pressure to electrical voltage.

Power. Rate at which work is done; rate at which energy is transferred.

Pressure. Force divided by area.

Probe. Transducer assembly.

Propagation. Progression or travel.

Propagation speed. Speed with which a wave moves through a medium.

Pulse. A brief excursion of a quantity from its normal value; a few cycles.

Pulsed mode. Mode of operation in which pulsed ultrasound is used.

Pulsed ultrasound. Ultrasound produced in pulse form by applying electrical pulses to the transducer.

Pulse duration. Time from start to finish of a pulse.

Pulse-echo diagnostic ultrasound. Ultrasound imaging in which pulses are reflected and used to produce a display.

Pulse repetition frequency. Number of pulses per unit time. Sometimes called pulse repetition rate.

Pulse repetition period. Time from the beginning of one pulse to the beginning of the next.

Quality factor. Operating frequency divided by bandwidth.

Radiation force. Steady force exerted on an object on which a sound beam is incident.

Range equation. Relationship between round-trip pulse travel time and distance to a reflector.

Rayl. Unit of impedance.

Real time. Imaging with a real-time display.

Real-time display. A display that continuously images moving structures.

Reflection. Portion of sound returned from a media boundary.

Reflection angle. Angle between reflected sound direction and line perpendicular to media boundary.

Reflector. Media boundary that produces a reflection; reflecting surface.

Refraction. Change of sound direction on passing from one medium to another.

Registration. Positioning of reflectors in the display.

Rejection. Eliminating smaller-amplitude voltage pulses.

Resonant frequency. Operating frequency.

Reverberation. Multiple reflections.

Scanning. Sweeping a sound beam to produce an image.

Scan converter. Device that stores a gray-scale image and allows it to be displayed on a television monitor.

Scan line. A line produced on a display by moving a spot (produced by an electron beam) across the face at constant speed.

Scattering. Diffusion or redirection of sound in several directions on encountering a particle suspension or a rough surface.

Schlieren. An acousto-optic system that displays a cross section of beam shape.

Sensitivity. Ability of an imaging system to detect weak reflections.

Shadowing. Reduction in reflection amplitude from reflectors that lie behind a strongly reflecting or attenuating structure.

Side lobes. Minor beams of sound traveling out in directions not included in the primary beam.

sin. Abbreviation for sine.

Sine. The sine of angle A in Figure A3.1 is the length of side a divided by the length of side c.

Snell's law. Relates incidence and transmission angles of refraction.

Sound. Traveling wave of acoustic variables.

Sound beam. The region of a medium that contains virtually all the sound produced by a transducer.

Spatial pulse length. Length of space over which a burst occurs.

Specular reflection. Reflection from a smooth boundary.

Speed. Displacement divided by time over which displacement occurs.

Stiffness. Property of a medium: applied pressure divided by fractional volume change produced by the pressure.

Strength. Nonspecific term referring to amplitude or intensity.

Temperature. Condition of a body that determines transfer of heat to or from other bodies.

Thermocouple. A device that converts temperature to a voltage.

Transducer. Device that converts energy from one form to another.

Transducer array. Transducer assembly containing more than one transducer element.

Transducer assembly. Transducer element and damping and matching materials assembled in a case.

Transducer element. Piece of piezoelectric material in a transducer assembly.

Transmission angle. Angle between transmitted sound direction and line perpendicular to media boundary.

Ultrasound. Sound of frequency greater than 20 kHz.

Ultrasound transducer. Device that converts electrical energy to ultrasound energy and vice versa.

Velocity. Speed with direction of motion specified.

Voltage pulse. Brief excursion of voltage from its normal value.

Wave. Traveling variation of wave variables.

Wavelength. Length of space over which a cycle occurs.

Wave variables. Things that are functions of space and time in a wave.

Work. Force multiplied by displacement.

Answers to Exercises in the Text

Chapter 1

1.2.1. pulses, ultrasound, reflections, image
1.2.2. ultrasound, tissues
1.2.3. acoustic, diagnostic
1.2.4. biological
1.2.5. a. 4; b. 3; c. 6; d. 1; e. 5; f. 2
1.2.6. a. 3; b. 1; c. 2

Chapter 2

2.2.1. wave variables
2.2.2. acoustic variables
2.2.3. 20,000
2.2.4. pressure, density, temperature, particle motion
2.2.5. c, d, e
2.2.6. a, e
2.2.7. cycles
2.2.8. hertz, Hz
2.2.9. time
2.2.10. reciprocal
2.2.11. space
2.2.12. wave
2.2.13. propagation speed, frequency

2.2.14. density, stiffness
2.2.15. e
2.2.16. 1540, 1.54, 1.54
2.2.17. e
2.2.18. a, c, b
2.2.19. 1.54
2.2.20. decreases
2.2.21. 10
2.2.22. higher
2.2.23. d
2.2.24. b
2.2.25. higher
2.2.26. mechanical longitudinal
2.2.27. doubled
2.2.28. 1
2.2.29. unchanged
2.2.30. energy
2.2.31. e
2.2.32. false
2.2.33. true

2.3.1. continuous wave
2.3.2. pulses
2.3.3. pulses
2.3.4. pulses
2.3.5. period
2.3.6. reciprocal
2.3.7. time
2.3.8. length, space
2.3.9. Duty factor
2.3.10. period
2.3.11. wavelength
2.3.12. 1
2.3.13. 6
2.3.14. 2
2.3.15. 1.3 (period is 0.33 μs)
2.3.16. 1
2.3.17. 0.0013

2.4.1. variation
2.4.2. power, area
2.4.3. W/cm²
2.4.4. amplitude
2.4.5. doubled
2.4.6. halved
2.4.7. unchanged
2.4.8. quadrupled

2.4.9. 5
2.4.10. peak, average
2.4.11. average, peak
2.4.12. b
2.4.13. a. 3; b. 1; c. 3
2.4.14. 2
2.4.15. 3

2.5.1. amplitude, intensity
2.5.2. absorption, reflection, scattering
2.5.3. length
2.5.4. dB, dB/cm
2.5.5. 1
2.5.6. 3 dB/cm
2.5.7. increases
2.5.8. doubled, doubled, quadrupled
2.5.9. unchanged
2.5.10. sound, heat
2.5.11. No (absorption is one part of attenuation)
2.5.12. Higher
2.5.13. 50, 1.5, 50, 1
2.5.14. density, propagation speed
2.5.15. increased
2.5.16. 5
2.5.17. attenuation coefficient
2.5.18. decreases
2.5.19. 0.32 (intensity ratio is 0.159), 1.5
2.5.20. 0.00000002
2.5.21. 1,540,000 (propagation speed is 1540 m/s)

2.6.1. a
2.6.2. e
2.6.3. a. 4; b. 1; c. 3; d. 5; e. 2
2.6.4. a. 2; b. 3; c. 4; d. 1
2.6.5. a. 3; b. 4; c. 1; d. 2; e. 5; f. 7; g. 6
2.6.6. a. 3; b. 4; c. 1; d. 2; e. 1; f. 3; g. 1; h. 5; i. 8; j. 7; k. 6; l. 9; m. 10
2.6.7. a. 1; b. 2, 3; c. 3; d. 1; e. 2
2.6.8. a. 1.54; b. 0.77; c. 3.1; d. 0.5; e. 2; f. 1; g. 0.002; h. 2; i. 2; j. 1.5; k. 6; l. 0.25; m. 0.25; n. 1; o. 125; p. 500; q. 1,630,000
2.6.9. c
2.6.10. a

3.2.1. impedances
3.2.2. impedances, intensity
3.2.3. impedances
3.2.4. 0.0008, 1.9992
3.2.5. 0.0002, 1.9998
3.2.6. 0.0008, 1.9992
3.2.7. 0.01 (incident intensity not needed)
3.2.8. 0.99
3.2.9. 20 (intensity ratio 0.01, use Table A4.1)
3.2.10. 0.01
3.2.11. 0 (impedances are the same)
3.2.12. 5, 0
3.2.13. True
3.2.14. False, in general (true only if propagation speeds are also equal)
3.2.15. scattering
3.2.16. False
3.2.17. 0.9990
3.2.18. air, reflection
3.2.19. 0.01
3.2.20. 0.43
3.2.21. d
3.2.22. True
3.2.23. False
3.2.24. a
3.2.25. True

3.3.1. direction
3.3.2. larger than, equal to
3.3.3. smaller than, equal to
3.3.4. equal to, equal to
3.3.5. 30, 20
3.3.6. 30, 30
3.3.7. 30, 41
3.3.8. 0.04 (incidence angle and intensity are not needed; the propagation speeds are equal, so that the calculation is the same as with normal incidence)
3.3.9. 0.2 (no refraction; calculate as with normal incidence)
3.3.10. normal incidence, media propagation speeds are equal
3.3.11. media propagation speeds are equal (no refraction)
3.3.12. density, propagation speed

3.3.13.   33

3.4.1.   frequency, motion
3.4.2.   higher
3.4.3.   lower
3.4.4.   equal to
3.4.5.   motion
3.4.6.   1.02
3.4.7.   0.026
3.4.8.   -0.026
3.4.9.   reflected, incident
3.4.10.   cosine
3.4.11.   1.01 (the cosine of 60 degrees is 0.5; the Doppler shift is cut in half)

3.5.1.   40 (20 attenuation, 20 reflection)
3.5.2.   0.0001
3.5.3.   0.0001, 0.00025
3.5.4.   0.00063, 0.00063

3.6.1.   pulses, echoes, display
3.6.2.   propagation speed, time
3.6.3.   4
3.6.4.   7
3.6.5.   7.7
3.6.6.   1
3.6.7.   reverberations
3.6.8.   e
3.6.9.   two

3.7.1.   sound travel, reflections
3.7.2.   spatial pulse length
3.7.3.   True
3.7.4.   1.5
3.7.5.   1
3.7.6.   2.3, 0.2
3.7.7.   halved
3.7.8.   doubled
3.7.9.   False
3.7.10.   False
3.7.11.   1
3.7.12.   10 (less than 10 MHz in many applications)
3.7.13.   wavelength, spatial pulse length
3.7.14.   attenuation

3.8.1.   True (longitudinal resolution = 0.3 mm)
3.8.2.   resolution, depth of penetration
3.8.3.   1, 10
3.8.4.   propagation speeds, equal

3.8.5. d

3.8.6. e

3.8.7. d

3.8.8. 0.04

3.8.9. 0.0001 (40 dB for 8-cm round trip, 20-dB reflection; number of cycles not needed)

3.8.10. 0.01 (6-dB attenuation for 6-cm round-trip path length; frequency is 1 MHz; 20-dB reflection)

3.8.11. impedances

3.8.12. densities, propagation speeds

Chapter 4

4.2.1. energy

4.2.2. electrical, ultrasound

4.2.3. piezoelectricity

4.2.4. discs

4.2.5. thickness

4.2.6. element, assembly

4.2.7. element, assembly

4.2.8. continuous-wave

4.2.9. pulses

4.2.10. decreases

4.2.11. cycles, longitudinal resolution, bandwidth, quality factor

4.2.12. efficiency, sensitivity

4.2.13. two, six

4.2.14. 0.2

4.2.15. 1

4.2.16. reflection

4.2.17. air

4.2.18. e

4.2.19. False

4.2.20. frequencies

4.3.1. 4

4.3.2. near, far

4.3.3. near-zone

4.3.4. frequency or wavelength, diameter, distance

4.3.5. transducer diameter, wavelength

4.3.6. transducer diameter, frequency

4.3.7. one-half

4.3.8. two

4.3.9. decreases

4.3.10. increases

4.3.11. 30

4.3.12. 4.5, 3, 6, 12

4.3.13. 60

4.3.14. 3, 6, 9

4.3.15. longer, smaller

4.3.16. 120

4.3.17. 9, 6, 9, 12

4.3.18. longer, smaller

4.3.19. quadruples

4.3.20. doubles

4.3.21. doubled

4.4.1. separation, reflections

4.4.2. beam diameter

4.4.3. c, d, f

4.4.4. True

4.4.5. True

4.4.6. False (only true near the transducer)

4.4.7. b, c, e, f

4.5.1. element

4.5.2. linear, two-dimensional or area, annular

4.5.3. switched, phased

4.5.4. a. 1; b. 2, 3; c. 2, 3; d. 3, 1, 2; e. 1, 2, 3

4.5.5. one

4.5.6. two

4.5.7. two

4.5.8. a. 1; b. 2; c. 2; d. 2

4.5.9. b

4.5.10. a

4.5.11. c

4.6.1. a. 4; b. 3; c. 2; d. 1

4.6.2. a, d

4.6.3. a. 5; b. 0.3; c. 141; d. 9.8; e. 6.5

4.6.4. c

4.6.5. one-half, near-zone

4.6.6. focal

4.6.7. 6.5 (frequency not needed)

4.6.8. 0.7 (diameter not needed)

4.6.9. True

4.6.10. False

4.6.11. focal

4.6.12. True

4.6.13. False

4.6.14. a. 1, 3; b. 2; c. 2; d. 1

4.6.15. a

4.6.16. e

4.6.17. a

4.6.18. b, c, d

5.2.1. pulser, transducer, receiver, display
5.2.2. a. 4; b. 1; c. 2; d. 3
5.2.3. a. 2; b. 2; c. 2, 3; d. 3; e. 1; f. 1; g. 2; h. 1, 2; i. 2, 3;
j. 2, 3; k. 1, 2, 3; l. 1, 2, 3; m. 2, 3; n. 2, 3; o. 2, 3; p. 2, 3
5.2.4. pulse
5.2.5. amplitude, intensity
5.2.6. a. 3; b. 5; c. 1; d. 2; e. 4

5.3.1. amplification, compensation, compression, demodulation, rejection
5.3.2. a. 2; b. 5; c. 3; d. 1; e. 4
5.3.3. 100, 10,000, 40
5.3.4. 1
5.3.5. 10
5.3.6. b, e
5.3.7. depth, distance
5.3.8. times
5.3.9. dynamic, demodulator, display
5.3.10. 2
5.3.11. pulses, voltages
5.3.12. False
5.3.13. a

5.4.1. A, B, M
5.4.2. a. 2, 9; b. 1, 3, 7, 8; c. 1, 3, 4, 6, 8; d. 3, 5, 9
5.4.3. cathode-ray
5.4.4. deflection
5.4.5. time, distance or depth
5.4.6. True
5.4.7. M
5.4.8. time, propagation speed
5.4.9. depth
5.4.10. scanning
5.4.11. 2.6
5.4.12. 77
5.4.13. gray-scale
5.4.14. scan converter

5.5.1. A, M
5.5.2. B, C
5.5.3. mechanical, electronic
5.5.4. frame
5.5.5. pulsed
5.5.6. lines, frame
5.5.7. 128
5.5.8. 2.6

5.5.9. No (25 × 200 × 20 = 100,000: greater than 77,000)

5.5.10. False (latter portion)

5.6.1. Doppler shift

5.6.2. False

5.6.3. one, two

5.6.4. frequencies

5.6.5. False

5.6.6. motion

5.6.7. gate

5.6.8. display

5.6.9. gate, voltage generator

5.6.10. depth

5.6.11. True

5.7.1. a. 1; b. 2, 3; c. 3; d. 3; e. 2, 3; f. 4, 5; g. 4, 5; h. 4; i. 2, 6

5.7.2. separation

5.7.3. weaker

5.7.4. b

5.7.5. d

5.7.6. True

5.7.7. b

5.7.8. c

5.7.9. False

5.7.10 e

5.7.11 a

5.8.1. a

5.8.2. b

5.8.3. d

5.8.4. c

5.8.5. a

5.8.6. b, f, e, d, c, a

5.8.7. a. 1, 3, 5; b. 2, 4, 6; c. 2, 4, 6; d. 1, 3, 6

5.8.8. d

5.8.9. d

5.8.10. a. 1, 2; b. 1, 2; c. 2, 3; d. 1, 2, 3; e. 2, 3; f. 1, 2, 3

5.8.11. reception

5.8.12. reflections or echoes

5.8.13. reflection

5.8.14. pulse-echo

5.8.15. strength, direction, time

5.8.16. shift

5.8.17. display, voltages or pulses

5.8.18. receiver

5.8.19. pulser

5.8.20. receiver

5.8.21. a

5.8.22. f

5.8.23.	b
5.8.24.	e
5.8.25.	c
5.8.26.	d
5.8.27.	c
5.8.28.	b
5.8.29.	a
5.8.30.	False

Chapter 6

6.2.1.	rods, water, alcohol
6.2.2.	a. 1; b. 2; c. 3; d. 6; e. 4; f. 3; g. 7; h. 7
6.2.3.	a. 5; b. 5; c. 4; d. 3; e. 2; f. 1; g. 1; h. 1
6.2.4.	True
6.2.5.	True
6.2.6.	1
6.3.1.	a. 4, 5, 6, 7; b. 4, 5, 6, 7; c. 1, 2; d. 3; e. 2
6.3.2.	a. 1; b. 2; c. 1; d. 2; e. 2
6.3.3.	transducer
6.3.4.	e
6.3.5.	a. 2; b. 1; c. 4; d. 5; e. 3
6.3.6.	a. 2, 12 or 1, 9; b. 3, 12; c. 3, 8; d. 4 or 2, 9; e. 1, 7; f. 5, 10; g. 6, 11
6.4.1.	d
6.4.2.	False
6.4.3.	b
6.5.1.	a. 2; b. 1, 2; c. 2, 3; d. 3; e. 3; f. 2, 3
6.5.2.	a. 2; b. 3; c. 1

Chapter 7

7.4.1.	False
7.4.2.	False
7.4.3.	b
7.4.4.	No
7.4.5.	Yes
7.4.6.	a
7.4.7.	a
7.4.8.	b
7.4.9.	e
7.4.10.	False

Chapter 8

8.1.	a
8.2.	c
8.3.	d
8.4.	e

8.5. e

8.6. a

8.7. e

8.8. c

8.9. c

8.10. False (only true near the transducer)

8.11. False (only true for normal incidence or oblique incidence when densities and propagation speeds of the media are equal)

8.12. False (see comment for 8.11)

8.13. c

8.14. d

8.15. e

8.16. r

8.17.

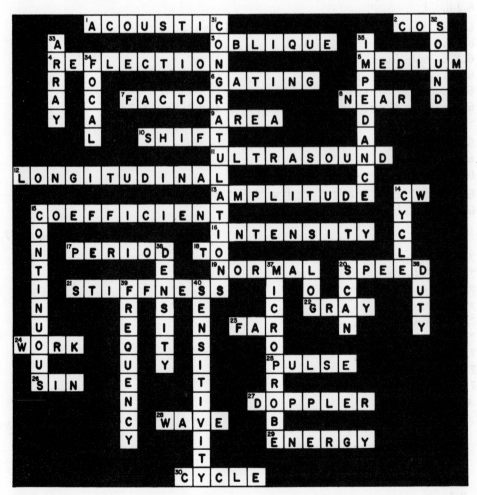

Appendixes

Appendix 1
Equations List

For convenient reference, equations presented throughout this book are compiled here. An asterisk indicates that the equation is specifically for soft tissues. Two asterisks indicate that the equation is specifically for normal incidence.

$$\text{period } (\mu s) = \frac{1}{\text{frequency (MHz)}}$$

$$\text{propagation speed (mm/}\mu s) = \text{frequency (MHz)} \times \text{wavelength (mm)}$$

$$\text{wavelength (mm)} = \frac{\text{propagation speed (mm/}\mu s)}{\text{frequency (MHz)}}$$

$$\overset{*}{=} \frac{1.54}{\text{frequency (MHz)}}$$

$$\text{pulse repetition period (ms)} = \frac{1}{\text{pulse repetition frequency (kHz)}}$$

$$\text{pulse duration } (\mu s) = \text{number of cycles in pulse} \times \text{period } (\mu s)$$

$$\text{duty factor} = \frac{\text{pulse duration } (\mu s)}{\text{pulse repetition period (ms)} \times 1000}$$

spatial pulse length (mm) = number of cycles in pulse ×
wavelength (mm)

$$\stackrel{*}{=} \frac{\text{number of cycles in pulse} \times 1.54}{\text{frequency (MHz)}}$$

$$\text{intensity (W/cm}^2) = \frac{\text{power (W)}}{\text{beam area (cm}^2)}$$

temporal average intensity (W/cm²) = duty factor ×
temporal peak intensity (W/cm²)

$$\text{SP/SA factor} = \frac{\text{spatial peak intensity (W/cm}^2)}{\text{spatial average intensity (W/cm}^2)}$$

attenuation (dB) = attenuation coefficient (dB/cm) ×
path length (cm) $\stackrel{*}{=}$ frequency (MHz) × path length (cm)

$$\text{depth of penetration (cm)} \stackrel{*}{=} \frac{3}{\text{attenuation coefficient (dB/cm)}}$$

$$\stackrel{*}{=} \frac{3}{\text{frequency (MHz)}}$$

impedance (rayl) = density (kg/m³) × propagation speed (m/s)

reflected intensity (W/cm²) $\stackrel{**}{=}$ incident intensity (W/cm²) ×
$$\left[\frac{\text{medium two impedance} - \text{medium one impedance}}{\text{medium two impedance} + \text{medium one impedance}}\right]^2$$

transmitted intensity (W/cm²) $\stackrel{**}{=}$ incident intensity (W/cm²) −
reflected intensity (W/cm²)

$$\text{intensity reflection coefficient} = \frac{\text{reflected intensity (W/cm}^2)}{\text{incident intensity (W/cm}^2)}$$

$$\stackrel{**}{=} \left[\frac{\text{medium two impedance} + \text{medium one impedance}}{\text{medium two impedance} + \text{medium one impedance}}\right]^2$$

$$\text{intensity transmission coefficient} = \frac{\text{transmitted intensity (W/cm}^2)}{\text{incident intensity (W/cm}^2)}$$

$$\stackrel{**}{=} 1 - \text{intensity reflection coefficient}$$

reflection angle (degrees) = incidence angle (degrees)

sine of transmission angle = sine of incidence angle ×
$$\left[\frac{\text{medium two propagation speed (mm/}\mu\text{s)}}{\text{medium one propagation speed (mm/}\mu\text{s)}}\right]$$

Doppler shift = reflected frequency (MHz)
− incident frequency (MHz)

$$= \pm \frac{2 \times \text{reflector speed (m/s)}}{\text{propagation speed (m/s)} + \text{reflector speed (m/s)}}$$

distance to reflector (mm) $\overset{*}{=}$ 0.77 × pulse round-trip time (μs)

$$\text{longitudinal resolution (mm)} \overset{*}{=} 0.77 \times \frac{\text{number of cycles in pulse}}{\text{frequency (MHz)}}$$

$$\text{operating frequency (MHz)} = \frac{\text{propagation speed (mm/μs)}}{2 \times \text{thickness (mm)}}$$

$$\text{quality factor} = \frac{\text{operating frequency (MHz)}}{\text{bandwidth (MHz)}}$$

near-zone length (mm) $\overset{*}{=}$

$$\frac{[\text{transducer diameter (mm)}]^2 \times \text{frequency (MHz)}}{6}$$

near-zone beam diameter (mm) $\overset{*}{=}$ transducer diameter (mm)

$$- \frac{3 \times \text{distance (mm)}}{\text{frequency (MHz)} \times \text{transducer diameter (mm)}}$$

far-zone beam diameter (mm) $\overset{*}{=}$

$$\frac{3 \times \text{distance (mm)}}{\text{frequency (MHz)} \times \text{transducer diameter (mm)}}$$

lateral resolution (mm) = beam diameter (mm)

$$\text{maximum depth (cm)} = \frac{77}{\text{maximum pulse repetition frequency (kHz)}}$$

maximum depth (cm) × lines per frame × frame rate = 77,000

Appendix 2
Physics Concepts

A2.1 Introduction

The terms discussed in this appendix are defined in the Glossary, and their units are given in Appendix 5. The definitions are amplified here, and the terms are related to one another.

A2.2 Force and Pressure

If there were no **forces**, everything would be in a state of rest or steady motion. Forces change the state of rest or motion of matter. When considering sound, the force divided by the area over which the force is applied is a useful quantity. This is called pressure. It is force per unit area (the concentration of force).

$$\text{pressure (N/m}^2) = \frac{\text{force (N)}}{\text{area (m}^2)}$$

A given force applied to an object may produce markedly different results if the pressures at which it is applied are different. If, for example, a small force is applied by a hand to an inflated toy balloon, the balloon will simply move. If the same small force is applied by a sharp needle, the balloon will break. The difference is that the needle applies the force over a very small area (a very high pressure), breaking the balloon.

Application of force or pressure changes the state of rest or motion of matter. Motion may be described in many ways.

Displacement is the distance that a body has moved.

Speed is the rate at which position is changing. It is the distance moved divided by the time over which the movement occurs.

$$\text{speed (m/s)} = \frac{\text{displacement (m)}}{\text{time (s)}}$$

Velocity is the same as speed except that the direction of motion is specified.

Acceleration is the rate at which velocity is changing. It is the change in velocity (change in speed or direction or both) divided by the time over which the change occurs.

$$\text{acceleration (m/s}^2) = \frac{\text{velocity change (m/s)}}{\text{time (s)}}$$

Mass is a measure of an object's resistance to acceleration. Weight is the gravitational force between two bodies attracting each other. The mass of a body is the same whether it is on the earth or on the moon, but the weights of the body in the two places are quite different.

Density is the concentration of mass. It is the mass divided by the volume taken up by the mass (mass per unit volume).

$$\text{density (kg/m}^3) = \frac{\text{mass (kg)}}{\text{volume (m}^3)}$$

Stiffness is a description of the resistance of a material to compression. It is equal to the applied pressure divided by the fractional change in volume resulting from the pressure.

$$\text{stiffness (N/m}^2) = \frac{\text{pressure (N/m}^2)}{\text{fractional volume change}}$$

The fractional volume change is the volume before the pressure was applied minus the volume after the pressure was applied, all divided by the volume before the pressure was applied.

If a material has high stiffness, little change in volume will occur when pressure is applied. If it has low stiffness, a large change in volume will occur when pressure is applied.

**A2.5
Law of
Motion**

Newton's second law of motion relates three of the things we have discussed in this appendix. It says that the force applied to a body is equal to the mass of the body multiplied by the acceleration of the body resulting from the applied force.

$$\text{force (N)} = \text{mass (kg)} \times \text{acceleration (m/s}^2)$$

If more than one force is applied, the net force (resulting from combination of the applied forces) is the force used in the equation. The acceleration will always be in the direction of the net force.

**A2.6
Work,
Energy,
and
Power**

Work is done when a force acts against a resistance to produce motion of a body. It is equal to the applied net force multiplied by the distance the body moves (displacement).

$$\text{work (J)} = \text{force (N)} \times \text{displacement (m)}$$

If there is no motion, no work is done. If a body is in motion but no force is being applied, again, no work is done.

Energy is the capability of doing work. A body must have energy in order to do work on another body. When a body does work, it loses energy. When a body has work done on it, it receives energy. Work may be thought of as the transfer of energy from one body (the one doing the work) to another (the one having work done on it). The energy transferred is equal to the work done.

Power is the rate at which work is done or the rate at which energy is transferred. It is equal to the work done divided by the time required to do the work. It is also equal to energy transferred divided by the time required to transfer the energy.

$$\text{power (W)} = \frac{\text{work (J)}}{\text{time (s)}} = \frac{\text{energy (J)}}{\text{time (s)}}$$

Heat is one type of energy. It is the energy due to thermal molecular motion.

Temperature is the condition of a body that determines transfer of heat to or from other bodies. No heat flows when two bodies of equal temperatures come in contact with each other. Heat flows from a body of higher temperature to one of lower temperature when they come in contact.

A2.1. Match the following:

a. pressure: _____   1. force $\times$ displacement
b. speed: _____   2. displacement change/time
c. acceleration: _____   3. mass $\times$ acceleration
d. density: _____   4. work/time
e. force: _____   5. force/area
f. stiffness: _____   6. velocity change/time
g. work: _____   7. mass/volume
h. power: _____   8. pressure/fractional volume
                                 change

A2.2. To convert speed to velocity, _____ must be specified.

A2.3. Heat is one type of _____.

A2.4. Pressure is the concentration of _____.

A2.5. Density is the concentration of _____.

A2.6. Speed is the rate at which _____ changes.

A2.7. Acceleration is the rate at which _____ changes.

A2.8. Newton's second law of motion states that _____ equals _____ times _____.

A2.9. Stiffness is a description of the resistance of a material to _____.

A2.10. Power is the rate at which _____ is done.

A2.11. Energy is the capability of doing _____

A2.12. Temperature is the condition of a body that determines transfer of _____ to or from other bodies.

A2.13. If a force of 50 N acts uniformly over an area of 20 m², the pressure is _____ N/m².

A2.14. If a body moves 50 m uniformly in 5 s, its speed is _____ m/s.

A2.15. If a body accelerates uniformly to the east at 5 m/s², its velocity 5 s after the starting from zero speed is _____ m/s east.

A2.16. Five kilograms of matter with a volume of 10 m³ have a density of _____ kg/m³.

A2.17. If a pressure of 5 N/m² changes the volume of a body from 0.5 m³ to 0.4 m³, the fractional volume change is _____ .

A2.18. The stiffness of the material of the body in Problem A2.17 is _____ N/m².

A2.19. A 5-kg mass subjected to a 15-N force west will have acceleration of _____ m/s² in the _____ direction.

A2.20. If a force of 3 N moves a body 4 m, the work done is _____ J.

A2.21. If the movement in Problem A2.20 occurs in 6 s, the power is _____ J/s or _____ W.

A2.22. In Problem A2.20, the energy transferred is _____ J.

Appendix 3
Algebra and Trigonometry

Only the basic concepts of algebra and trigonometry that are applicable to the material in this book will be considered in this appendix.

A3.1 Introduction

Transposition of quantities in algebraic equations is accomplished by performing identical mathematical operations on both sides.

A3.2 Algebra

For the equation

$$x + y = z$$

Example A3.2.1

transpose to get x alone (solve for x). To do this, subtract y from both sides:

$$x + y - y = z - y$$

Since $y - y = 0$; the left-hand side of the equation is

$$x + y - y = x + 0 = x$$

so that

$$x = z - y$$

175

Example A3.2.2 For the equation

$$x - y = z$$

solve for x. Add y to both sides:

$$x - y + y = z + y$$
$$x + 0 = z + y$$
$$x = z + y$$

Example A3.2.3 For the equation

$$xy = z$$

solve for x. Divide both sides by y:

$$\frac{xy}{y} = \frac{z}{y}$$

Since $\frac{y}{y} = 1$;

$$\frac{xy}{y} = x(1) = x$$

and

$$x = \frac{z}{y}$$

Example A3.2.4 For the equation

$$\frac{x}{y} = z$$

solve for x. Multiply both sides by y:

$$\frac{x}{y} y = zy$$
$$x(1) = zy$$
$$x = zy$$

Using some numbers, and combining the previous examples, consider the equation

$$\frac{5x + 3}{2} - 3 = 1$$

Solve for x. Add 3:

$$\frac{5x + 3}{2} - 3 + 3 = 1 + 3$$

$$\frac{5x + 3}{2} = 4$$

Multiply by 2:

$$\frac{5x + 3}{2} \times 2 = 4 \times 2$$

$$5x + 3 = 8$$

Subtract 3:

$$5x + 3 - 3 = 8 - 3$$
$$5x = 5$$

Divide by 5:

$$x = 1$$

Substitution of the answer into the original equation shows that the equality holds:

$$\frac{5(1) + 3}{2} - 3 = 1$$

$$\frac{8}{2} - 3 = 1$$

$$4 - 3 = 1$$
$$1 = 1$$

Example
A3.2.6

For the equation

$$\text{propagation speed} = \text{frequency} \times \text{wavelength}$$

solve for wavelength. Divide by frequency:

$$\frac{\text{propagation speed}}{\text{frequency}} = \frac{\text{frequency} \times \text{wavelength}}{\text{frequency}}$$

$$\frac{\text{propagation speed}}{\text{frequency}} = \text{wavelength}$$

Example
A3.2.7

If the intensity reflection coefficient is 0.1 and the reflected intensity is 5 mW/cm², find the incident intensity, given that

$$\text{intensity reflection coefficient} = \frac{\text{reflected intensity}}{\text{incident intensity}}$$

Multiply by incident intensity:

$$\text{intensity reflected coefficient} \times \text{incident intensity} =$$
$$\frac{\text{reflected intensity}}{\text{incident intensity}} \times \text{incident intensity} = \text{reflected intensity}$$

Divide by intensity reflection coefficient:

$$\frac{\text{intensity reflection coefficient} \times \text{incident intensity}}{\text{intensity reflection coefficient}} =$$
$$\frac{\text{reflected intensity}}{\text{intensity reflection coefficient}}$$

$$\text{incident intensity} = \frac{\text{reflected intensity}}{\text{intensity reflection coefficient}}$$

$$= \frac{5 \text{ mW/cm}^2}{0.1}$$

$$= 50 \text{ mW/cm}^2$$

If the intensity reflection coefficient is 0.01 and the medium one impedance is 4.5, find the medium two impedance, given that

$$\text{intensity reflection coefficient} =$$
$$\left[\frac{\text{medium two impedance} - \text{medium one impedance}}{\text{medium two impedance} + \text{medium one impedance}}\right]^2$$

Take the square root of each side:

$$\frac{(\text{intensity reflection coefficient})^{\frac{1}{2}}}{\frac{\text{medium two impedance} - \text{medium one impedance}}{\text{medium two impedance} + \text{medium one impedance}}}$$

Multiply by the sum of medium two impedance and medium one impedance:

$$(\text{intensity reflection coefficient})^{\frac{1}{2}} \times$$
$$(\text{medium two impedance} + \text{medium one impedance}) =$$
$$\text{medium two impedance} - \text{medium one impedance}$$

Add the medium one impedance:

$$(\text{intensity reflection coefficient})^{\frac{1}{2}} \times$$
$$(\text{medium two impedance} + \text{medium one impedance}) +$$
$$\text{medium one impedance} = \text{medium two impedance}$$

Subtract (intensity reflection coefficient)$^{\frac{1}{2}}$ × medium two impedance:

$$[(\text{intensity reflection coefficient})^{\frac{1}{2}} \times \text{medium one impedance}]$$
$$+ \text{medium one impedance} = \text{medium two impedance}$$
$$- [(\text{intensity reflection coefficient})^{\frac{1}{2}} \times \text{medium two impedance}]$$

$$\text{medium one impedance} [1 + (\text{intensity reflection coefficient})^{\frac{1}{2}}]$$
$$= \text{medium two impedance} [1 - (\text{intensity reflection coefficient})^{\frac{1}{2}}]$$

Divide by [1 − (intensity reflection coefficient)^{½}] and interchange sides of the equation:

$$\text{medium two impedance} = \text{medium one impedance}$$
$$\left[\frac{1 + (\text{intensity reflection coefficient})^{½}}{1 - (\text{intensity reflection coefficient})^{½}}\right]$$
$$= 4.5 \left[\frac{1 + (0.01)^{½}}{1 - (0.01)^{½}}\right]$$
$$= 4.5 \left[\frac{1 + 0.1}{1 - 0.1}\right] = 4.5 \left[\frac{1.1}{0.9}\right]$$
$$= 4.5 \, (1.22) = 5.5$$
$$\text{medium two impedance} = 5.5$$

Example A3.2.9 A sonographer is twice as old as her diagnostic instrument was when she was as old as it is now. She is 24 years old. How old is the instrument? Let x = the instrument's present age. Let y = the instrument's age when the sonographer's age was x. The sonographer's present age is $24 = 2y$. Let z = years since the sonographer's age was x and the instrument's age was y. From the information given, we have

$$y + z = x$$
$$x + z = 24$$
$$2y = 24$$

Now solve these three equations for x:

$$y = 24/2 = 12$$
$$z = 24 - x$$
$$x = y + z = 12 + 24 - x$$
$$2x = 36$$
$$x = 18$$

The instrument is 18 years old. It is time to replace the instrument, but not the sonographer.

A3.2.1. Solve each of the following for x:

    a. $x + y + 2 = z$

    b. $x - y = z - 1$

    c. $2xy = z$

    d. $x/y = 3z$

    e. $\dfrac{x + 5}{4} - 2 = 4$

    f. $\dfrac{3x + 3}{2} - 2 = 4$

A3.2.2. Solve each of the following for the quantity with the asterisk:

    a. propagation speed = frequency* × wavelength

    b. intensity = $\dfrac{\text{power}}{\text{beam area*}}$

    c. period = $\dfrac{1}{\text{frequency*}}$

A3.3
Trigonometry

If the sides and angles of a right triangle (one of the angles equals 90 degrees) are labeled as in Figure A3.1, the sine of angle A (sin A) and the cosine of angle A (cos A) are defined as follows:

$$\sin A = \frac{\text{length of side a}}{\text{length of side c}}$$

$$\cos A = \frac{\text{length of side b}}{\text{length of side c}}$$

Example A3.3.1

If the lengths of sides a, b, and c are 1, $\sqrt{3}$, and 2, respectively, what are sin A and cos A?

$$\sin A = \frac{1}{2} = 0.50$$

$$\cos A = \frac{\sqrt{3}}{2} = 0.87$$

If the sine or cosine is known, angle A may be found using a calculator or a table such as Table A3.1.

Example A3.3.2

If sin A is 0.5, what is A? From Table A3.1, A = 30 degrees.

Example A3.3.3

If cos A is 0.87, what is A? From Table A3.1, A = 30 degrees.

If angle A is known, sin A or cos A may be found using a calculator or a table such as Table A3.1.

Example A3.3.4

If A = 40 degrees, what are sin A and cos A? From Table A3.1, sin A = 0.64 and cos A = 0.77.

Exercises

A3.3.1. If sides a, b, and c in Figure A3.1 have lengths 3, 4, and 5, respectively, sin A is _____ and cos A is _____.

A3.3.2. If angle A is 90 degrees, sin A is _____ and cos A is _____.

A3.3.3. If sin A is 0.17, angle A is _____ degrees.

A3.3.4. If cos A is 0.94, angle A is _____ degrees.

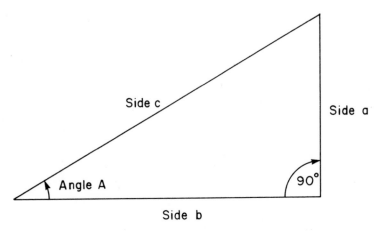

Figure A3.1. Sides and angles of a right triangle.

Table A3.1
Sines and Cosines for Various Angles

Angle A (degrees)	sin A	cos A
0	0.00	1.00
1	0.02	1.00
2	0.03	1.00
3	0.05	1.00
4	0.07	1.00
5	0.09	1.00
6	0.10	0.99
7	0.12	0.99
8	0.14	0.99
9	0.16	0.99
10	0.17	0.98
20	0.34	0.94
30	0.50	0.87
40	0.64	0.77
50	0.77	0.64
60	0.87	0.50
70	0.94	0.34
80	0.98	0.17
90	1.00	0.00

Appendix 4
Logarithms and Decibels

A4.1
Logarithms

The **logarithm** (log) (to the base 10) of a number is equal to one plus the number of times 10 must be multiplied by itself to result in that number.

Example
A4.1.1

What is the logarithm of 1000? To obtain 1000, 10 must be multiplied by itself two times:

$$10 \times 10 \times 10 = 1000$$

One plus two equals three, which then is equal to the logarithm (log) of 1000.

$$\log 1000 = 3$$

The logarithm of the reciprocal of a number is equal to the negative of the logarithm of the number.

What is the logarithm of 0.01?

$$0.01 = \frac{1}{100}$$

$$\log 100 = 2$$

$$\log 0.01 = \log \frac{1}{100} = -2$$

A4.1.1. The logarithm of 10 is _____.

A4.1.2. The logarithm of 0.1 is _____.

A4.1.3. The logarithm of 100 is _____.

A4.1.4. The logarithm of 0.001 is _____.

Decibels are units that result from taking 10 times the logarithm of the ratio of two powers or intensities.

A4.2
Decibels

Compare the following two powers in decibels: power one = 1 W; power two = 10 W.

$$10 \log \frac{\text{power one}}{\text{power two}} = 10 \log \frac{1}{10}$$

$$= 10 \ (-\log 10) = 10 \ (-1) = -10 \text{ dB}$$

Power one is 10 dB less than power two, or power one is 10 dB below power two. Also

$$10 \log \frac{\text{power two}}{\text{power one}} = 10 \log \frac{10}{1}$$

$$= 10 \ (\log 10) = 10 \ (1) = 10 \text{ dB}$$

Power two is 10 dB more than power one, or power two is 10 dB above power one.

Example An amplifier has a power output of 100 mW when the input power is
A4.2.2 0.1 mW. What is the amplifier gain in decibels?

$$\text{amplifier gain (dB)} = 10 \log \frac{\text{power out}}{\text{power in}}$$

$$= 10 \log \frac{100}{0.1} = 10 \log 1000 = 10 \ (3) = 30 \text{ dB}$$

Example An attenuator has a power output of 0.01 mW when the input power is
A4.2.3 100 mW. What is the attenuator attenuation in decibels?

$$\text{attenuator attenuation (dB)} = -10 \log \frac{\text{power out}}{\text{power in}}$$

$$= -10 \log \frac{0.01}{100} = -10 \log \frac{1}{10,000}$$

$$= -10 \ (-\log 10,000) = -10 \ (-4\ ) = 40 \text{ dB}$$

The first minus sign is used here to give the attenuation as a positive
number. If the minus number had not been used, we would have calculated the "gain" of the attenuator, which would have turned out to
be −40 dB. A gain of −40 dB is the same as an attenuation of 40 dB.

Example Compare intensity two with intensity one: intensity one = 10
A4.2.4 mW/cm²; intensity two = 0.01 mW/cm².

$$10 \log \frac{\text{intensity two}}{\text{intensity one}} = 10 \log \frac{0.01}{10}$$

$$= 10 \log \frac{1}{1000} = 10 \ (-\log 1000) = 10 \ (-3) = -30 \text{ dB}$$

Intensity two is 30 dB less than or below intensity one.

Example As sound passes through a medium, its intensity at one point is 1
A4.2.5 mW/cm² and at a point 10 cm farther along is 0.1 mW/cm². What are
the attenuation and attenuation coefficient? (See Section 2.5.)

$$\text{attenuation (dB)} = -10 \log \frac{\text{intensity at second point}}{\text{intensity at first point}}$$

$$= -10 \log \frac{0.1}{1} = -10 \log \frac{1}{10} = -10 \ (-\log 10)$$

$$= -10 \ (-1) = 10 \text{ dB}$$

Table A4.1

Decibel Values of Gain or Attenuation for Various
Values of Power or Intensity Ratio*

dB Gain or attenuation	Power or Intensity Ratio	
	Attenuation	Gain
0.1	0.977	1.02
0.2	0.955	1.05
0.3	0.933	1.07
0.4	0.912	1.10
0.5	0.891	1.12
0.6	0.871	1.15
0.7	0.851	1.17
0.8	0.832	1.20
0.9	0.813	1.23
1.0	0.794	1.26
2.0	0.631	1.58
3.0	0.501	1.99
4.0	0.398	2.51
5.0	0.316	3.16
6.0	0.251	3.98
7.0	0.200	5.01
8.0	0.159	6.31
9.0	0.126	7.94
10.0	0.100	10.00

*The ratio is output power or intensity divided by input power or intensity. In the case of
attenuation, it is the fraction of power or intensity remaining. For other dB values, add dB
and multiply ratios. For example, the power or intensity ratio (attenuation) for 36.5 dB
(0.5 + 6 + 10 + 10 + 10) is 0.891 × 0.251 × 0.1 × 0.1 × 0.1 = 0.000224.

See example A4.2.3 for comment on the first minus sign. The attenuation coefficient is the attenuation (dB) divided by the separation between the two points:

$$\text{attenuation coefficient (dB/cm)} = \frac{\text{attenuation (dB)}}{\text{separation (cm)}}$$

$$= \frac{10 \text{ dB}}{10 \text{ cm}} = 1 \text{ dB/cm}$$

Table A4.1 lists various values of power or intensity ratio with corresponding decibel values of gain or attenuation.

Exercises

A4.2.1. One watt is _____ dB below 100 W.

A4.2.2. One watt is _____ dB above 100 mW.

A4.2.3. If the input power is 1 mW and the output is 10,000 mW, the gain is _____ . dB.

A4.2.4. If the input power is 1 W and the output is 100 mW, the gain is _____ dB. The attenuation is _____ dB.

A4.2.5. If the intensities of traveling sound are 10 mW/cm² and 0.1 mW/cm² at two points 5 cm apart, the attenuation between the two points is _____ dB. The attenuation coefficient is _____ dB/cm.

A4.2.6. If an amplifier has a gain of 15 dB, the ratio of output power to input power is _____. (Use Table A4.1.)

A4.2.7. If an attenuator has an attenuation of 23.4 dB, the ratio of output power to input power is _____. (Use Table A4.1.1)

A4.2.8. If the intensity at the start of a path is 3 mW/cm² and the attenuation over the path is 1.9 dB, the intensity at the end of the path is _____ mW/cm². (Use Table A4.1.)

A4.2.9. If the output of a 22-dB gain amplifier is connected to the input of a 23-dB gain amplifier, the total gain is _____ dB. The overall power ratio is _____. (Use Table A4.1.)

A4.2.10. If a 17-dB attenuator is connected to a 15-dB amplifier, the overall gain is _____ dB. The overall attenuation is _____ dB. For a 1-W input, the output is _____ W. (Use Table A4.1.)

Appendix 5
Units

Units for the physics and acoustics quantities discussed in this book are presented in this appendix. They are drawn primarily from the international system of units (SI).

A5.1 Introduction

Units for the quantities discussed in this book are listed in Table A5.1. Equivalent units are given in Table A5.2. Prefixes for units are listed in Table A5.3, and conversion factors between common units are in Table A5.4.

A5.2 Tabulation

In algebraic equations involving units listed in the preceding section, the units for the quantity solved for are determined by manipulation of the units for the other quantities in the equation.

A5.3 Manipulation

Table A5.1

Units and Unit Symbols for Physics and Acoustics Quantities

Quantity	Unit	Unit symbol
Acceleration	meters/second²	m/s²
Angle	degrees	degrees
Area	meters²	m²
Attenuation	decibels*	dB
Attenuation coefficient	decibels/meter	dB/m
Beam area	meters²	m²
Pulse duration	seconds	s
Pulse repetition frequency	hertz	Hz
Pulse repetition period	seconds	s
Cosine	unitless	–
Density	kilograms/meter³	kg/m³
Depth of penetration	meters	m
Displacement	meters	m
Doppler shift	hertz	Hz
Duty factor	unitless	–
Energy	joules	J
Force	newtons	N
Fractional volume change	unitless	–
Frequency	hertz	Hz
Gain	decibels*	dB
Heat	joules	J
Impedance	rayls	–
Intensity	watts/meter²	W/m²
Intensity reflection coefficient	unitless	–
Intensity transmission coefficient	unitless	–
Mass	kilograms	kg
Period	seconds	s
Power	watts	W
Pressure	newtons/meter²	N/m²
Propagation speed	meters/second	m/s
Sine	unitless	–
Spatial pulse length	meters	m
Speed	meters/second	m/s
Stiffness	newtons/meter²	N/m²
SP/SA factor	unitless	–
Temperature	kelvins	K
Time	seconds	s
Velocity	meters/second	m/s
Voltage	volts	V
Volume	meters³	m³
Wavelength	meters	m
Work	joules	J

*See Appendix 4 for a discussion of decibels.

Table A5.2
Equivalent Units for Physics and Acoustics Quantities

Unit given in Table A5.1	Equivalent unit	Equivalent unit symbol
Hertz	1/second	1/s
Joules	newton-meters	N-m
Joules	watt-seconds	W-s
Rayls	kilograms/meter^2-second	kg/m^2-s
Newtons	kilogram-meters/second^2	kg-m/s^2
Newtons/meter^2	pascals	Pa
Watts	joules/second	J/s

Table A5.3
Unit Prefixes

Prefix	Factor*	Symbol
mega	1,000,000	M
kilo	1,000	k
centi	0.01	c
milli	0.001	m
micro	0.000001	μ

*Factor is the number of unprefixed units in a unit with the prefix. For example, there are 1,000 Hz in 1 kHz, and there is 0.001 m in 1 mm.

Table A5.4

Conversion Factors among Common Units

To convert	from	to	multiply by
Area	m²	cm²	10,000
	cm²	m²	0.0001
Attenuation	dB	Np (neper)	0.12
Displacement	m	mm	1,000
	m	cm	100
	m	km	0.001
	mm	m	0.001
	mm	km	0.000001
	km	mm	1,000,000
Frequency	Hz	kHz	0.001
	Hz	MHz	0.000001
	kHz	MHz	0.001
	MHz	kHz	1,000
	kHz	Hz	1,000
	MHz	Hz	1,000,000
Intensity	W/cm²	W/m²	10,000
	W/cm²	kW/m²	10
	W/cm²	mW/cm²	1,000
	W/m²	W/cm²	0.0001
	W/m²	mW/cm²	0.1
	W/m²	kW/m²	0.001
Speed	m/s	km/s	0.001
	km/s	m/s	1,000
	km/s	mm/μs	1

Determine the unit for frequency in the equation

$$\text{frequency} = \frac{\text{propagation speed (m/s)}}{\text{wavelength (m)}}$$

The units on the right-hand side of the equation are

$$\frac{\text{m/s}}{\text{m}} = 1/\text{s}$$

From Table A5.2, we find that

$$1/\text{s} = \text{Hz}$$

Therefore the frequency unit is hertz.

Determine the unit for frequency in the equation

$$\text{frequency} = \frac{\text{propagation speed (m/s)}}{\text{wavelength (mm)}}$$

The units on the right-hand side of the equation are

$$\frac{\text{m/s}}{\text{mm}}$$

From Table A5.3, we find that 1 mm equals 0.001 m, so that

$$\frac{\text{m/s}}{0.001 \text{ m}} = 1000 \ 1/\text{s}$$

and from Tables A5.2 and A5.3,

$$1000 \ 1/\text{s} = 1000 \text{ Hz} = 1 \text{ kHz}$$

Therefore the frequency unit is kilohertz. To convert a frequency given in kilohertz to megahertz, multiply by 0.001. To convert a frequency given in kilohertz to hertz, multiply by 1000.

Determine the unit for intensity in the equation

$$\text{intensity} = \frac{\text{power (W)}}{\text{area (cm}^2)}$$

The units on the right-hand side of the equation are

$$\frac{\text{W}}{\text{cm}^2}$$

Therefore the intensity unit is watts per centimeter squared.

Example A5.3.4 — Determine the unit for impedance in the equation

$$\text{impedance} = \text{density (kg/m}^3) \times \text{propagation speed (km/s)}$$

The units on the right-hand side of the equation are

$$\frac{kg}{m^3} \times \frac{km}{s}$$

From Table A5.3,

$$\frac{kg}{m^3} \times \frac{km}{s} = \frac{kg}{m^3} \times \frac{1000 \text{ m}}{s} = 1000 \; \frac{kg}{m^2\text{-}s}$$

From Table A5.2,

$$1000 \; \frac{kg}{m^2\text{-}s} = 1000 \text{ rayl}$$

From Table A5.3,

$$1000 \text{ rayl} = 1 \text{ krayl}$$

Therefore the impedance unit is kilorayl. Since this is uncommon, it would be better to multiply the answer by 1000 to give the result in rayls.

Exercises

A5.1. The unit of frequency in the equation

$$\text{frequency} = \frac{\text{propagation speed (km/s)}}{\text{wavelength (mm)}}$$

is _____. To convert frequency in this unit to frequency in kilohertz, multiply by _____.

A5.2. A frequency of 50 kHz is equal to _____ MHz and _____ Hz.

A5.3. A speed of 1.5 mm/μs is equal to _____ km/s, _____ m/s, _____ cm/s, and _____ mm/s.

A5.4. If the frequency is 2 MHz and

$$\text{period} = \frac{1}{\text{frequency}}$$

the period is _____ μs, _____ ms, or _____ s.

A.5.5 Mass is given in units of
  a. megahertz
  b. kilogram
  c. telegram
  d. millinery
  e. none of the above

A5.6. Displacement is given in
  a. megahertz
  b. megaphone
  c. centipede
  d. meter
  e. all of the above

A5.7. Attenuation is given in
  a. decimal
  b. decimate
  c. decibel
  d. decimeter
  e. decihertz

Appendix 6
Common Misconceptions

Some errors that have been observed to appear frequently in ultrasound literature are listed in this appendix.

1. "Propagation speed increases with density." If two media have the same stiffness, the one with greater density will have a similar propagation speed (Section 2.2).
2. "Reflections are produced by density differences." With normal incidence, reflections are produced by impedance changes (changes in density or stiffness or both) (Section 3.2). With oblique incidence, reflections are produced by changes in impedance or propagation speed or both (changes in density or stiffness or both) (Section 3.3).
3. "Absence of reflection means that media impedances are the same." This is true only with normal incidence. With oblique incidence, it is possible for there to be no reflection even when media impedances are different (Section 3.3).
4. "Snell's law states that the angle of incidence equals the angle of reflection." These angles are equal, but this is not Snell's law. It states that the sine of the transmission angle divided by the sine of the incidence angle equals the medium two propagation speed divided by the medium one propagation speed (Section 3.3).

5. "In the near zone, the beam diameter for a disc transducer is equal to the disc diameter." Beam diameter decreases as the distance from the transducer is increased out to the near-zone length (Section 4.3).

6. "An echo-free region on a display is a translucent or transonic region." The region should be called echo-free or anechoic. Translucent or transonic means that the ultrasound passes through the area uninhibited. This is true only if attenuation is low. Absence of echoes does not guarantee this (Section 2.5).

Exercises

A6.1. Propagation speed increases with increasing
    a. stiffness
    b. density
    c. absorption
    d. attenuation
    e. both a and b

A6.2. Reflections are produced by changes in
    a. stiffness
    b. density
    c. absorption
    d. attenuation
    e. both a and b

A6.3. If no reflection occurs at a boundary, this always means that media impedances are equal in the case of
    a. normal incidence
    b. oblique incidence
    c. refraction
    d. both a and b
    e. both b and c

A6.4. If the propagation speeds in two media are equal, Snell's law states that the incidence angle equals the
    a. reflection angle
    b. transmission angle
    c. Doppler angle
    d. both a and b
    e. both b and c

A6.5. At a distance of one near-zone length from a disc transducer, the beam diameter is equal to the disc diameter divided by
    a. one
    b. two
    c. three
    d. pi
    e. one-fourth

A6.6. An echo-free region on a display is
  a. translucent
  b. transonic
  c. anechoic
  d. both a and b
  e. both b and c

Answers to Exercises in the Appendixes

A2.1. a. 5; b. 2; c. 6; d. 7; e. 3; f. 8; g. 1; h. 4
A2.2. direction
A2.3. energy
A2.4. force
A2.5. mass
A2.6. position
A2.7. velocity
A2.8. force, mass, acceleration
A2.9. compression
A2.10. work
A2.11. work
A2.12. heat
A2.13. 2.5
A2.14. 10
A2.15. 25
A2.16. 0.5
A2.17. 0.2 (pressure is not needed for the calculation)
A2.18. 25
A2.19. 3, west

A2.20. 12
A2.21. 2, 2
A2.22. 12

Appendix 3

A3.2.1. a. $z - y - 2$; b. $y + z - 1$; c. $z/2y$; d. $3yz$; e. 19; f. 3
A3.2.2. a. propagation speed/wavelength; b. power/intensity;
c. 1/period
A3.3.1. 0.6, 0.8
A3.3.2. 1, 0
A3.3.3. 10
A3.3.4. 20

Appendix 4

A4.1.1. 1
A4.1.2. -1
A4.1.3. 2
A4.1.4. -3
A4.2.1. 20
A4.2.2. 10
A4.2.3. 40
A4.2.4. -10, 10
A4.2.5. 20, 4
A4.2.6. 31.6
A4.2.7. 0.0046
A4.2.8. 1.94
A4.2.9. 45, 31,600
A4.2.10. -2, 2, 0.631

Appendix 5

A5.1. megahertz, 1000
A5.2. 0.05, 50,000
A5.3. 1.5, 1500, 150,000, 1,500,000
A5.4. 0.5, 0.0005, 0.0000005
A5.5. b
A5.6. d
A5.7. c

A6.1. a
A6.2. e
A6.3. a
A6.4. b
A6.5. b
A6.6. c

References

1. Powis RL: Ultrasound Physics . . . for the Fun of It. Denver, Unirad, 1978
2. Wells PNT: Biomedical Ultrasonics. New York, Academic, 1977
3. McDicken WN: Diagnostic Ultrasonics: Principles and Use of Instruments. New York, Wiley, 1976
4. Hussey M: Diagnostic Ultrasound: An Introduction to the Interactions between Ultrasound and Biological Tissues. New York, Wiley, 1975
5. Goss SA, Johnson RL, Dunn F: Comprehensive compilation of empirical ultrasonic properties of mammalian tissues. J Acoust Soc Am 64:423–457, 1978
6. Carson PL, Fischella PR, Oughton TV: Ultrasonic power and intensities produced by diagnostic ultrasound equipment. Ultrasound Med Biol 3:341–350, 1978
7. Yeh E: Reverberations in echocardiograms. J Clin Ultrasound 5:84–86, 1977
8. Skolnick ML, Meire HB, Lecky JW: Common artifacts in ultrasound scanning. J Clin Ultrasound 3:273–280, 1975
9. Hall AJ, Fleming JEE, Morley P, Barnett E: Technical pitfalls in ultrasonic B scan examinations. Med Biol Eng 10:631–642, 1972
10. Standard 100 millimeter test object. Reflections 1:74–91, 1975

11. Christensen SL, Carson PL: Performance survey of ultrasound instrumentation and feasibility of routine monitoring. Radiology, 122:449–454, 1977

12. Lopez H, Smith SW: Quality assurance testing of an ultrasound B-scanner with the AIUM test object. Medical Ultrasound 2:19–26, 1978

13. Hellman LM, Duffus GM, Donald I, Sunden B: Safety of diagnostic ultrasound in obstetrics. Lancet 1:1133–1135, 1970

14. Ziskin MC: Survey of patient exposure to diagnostic ultrasound, in Reid JM, Sikov MR (eds): Interaction of Ultrasound and Biological Tissues. DHEW publication (FDA) 73-8008 BRH/DBE 73-1. Rockville, Md, US Food and Drug Administration, 1972, pp 203–205

15. Taylor KJW: Current status of toxicity investigations. J Clin Ultrasound 2:149–156, 1974

16. Ulrich WD: Ultrasound dosage for nontherapeutic use on human beings—extrapolations from a literature survey. IEEE Trans Biomed Eng BME-21:48–51, 1974

17. Wells PNT: The possibility of harmful biological effects in ultrasonic diagnosis, in Reneman RS (ed): Cardiovascular Applications of Ultrasound. New York, American Elsevier, 1974

18. Hazzard DG: Symposium on Biological Effects and Characterizations of Ultrasound Sources. DHEW publication (FDA) 78-8048. Rockville, Md, US Food and Drug Administration, 1977

19. Nyborg, WL: Physical Mechanisms for Biological Effects of Ultrasound. DHEW publication (FDA) 78-8062. Rockville, Md, US Food and Drug Administration, 1977

20. Statement on mammalian in vivo ultrasonic biological effects. J Clin Ultrasound 5:2–4, 1977; Reflections 4:311, 1978

21. Who's Afraid of a Hundred Milliwatts per Square Centimeter (100 mW/cm²) SPTA? Oklahoma City, American Institute of Ultrasound in Medicine, 1979

22. Acoustical Terminology. USA standard ANSI S1.1-1960 (R-1976). New York, American National Standards Institute, 1960

Index

Absorption, 21, 146
Acceleration, 146, 171, 172, 190
Acoustic output of instruments, 83
  measurement of, 120, 124–126,
    141
Acoustic propagation, 2, 146, 151
Acoustics, 146
Acoustic variables, 5, 8, 140, 146
  and amplitude, 17
Acousto-optics, 124, 141, 146
Air, impedance of, 59
Algebra, 175–181
American Institute of Ultrasound in
    Medicine (AIUM)
  advice on safety considerations,
    137
  100-mm test object, 121, 141
  statement on ultrasonic bioeffects,
    133
A-mode operation. *See* Amplitude-
    mode operation
Amplification, 85, 91, 146
Amplifier, 85, 146
Amplitude, 5, 17, 140, 146
  attenuation of, 21, 22
  pulse, 82
Amplitude-mode (A-mode) operation,
    93, 96–98, 146
Anechoic region, 197
Angle
  cosine of, 40, 147, 182, 183, 190
  incidence, 32, 34–37, 149, 196

reflection, 34, 35, 151, 196
sine of, 35, 152, 182, 183, 190
transmission, 34, 35, 153, 196
units, 190
Angular resolution, 70
Annular array, 72, 146
Area
  beam, 17–18, 63, 147, 190
  unit conversion factors for, 192
  units, 190
Arrays, 72–74, 141, 153
  annular, 72, 146
  linear, 72–74, 150
    phased, 70, 72, 74, 105, 150
    switched, 72, 73, 105, 150
Artifacts, 109–113, 141
Attenuation, 21–24, 140, 147, 187
  combined with reflection, 41–44
  compensation of, 21, 85, 87
  and frequency, 50
  unit conversion factors for, 192
  units, 190
Attenuation coefficient, 21–24, 147
  units, 190
Axial resolution, 47
Azimuthal resolution, 70

Backscatter, 32, 66, 147
Balance, to measure radiation force,
    125
Ball suspension, to measure radiation
    force, 125

Bandwidth, 59, 147
Beam(s), sound, 61–66, 141, 152
    focusing of. *See* Focus or focusing
    unfocused, 21
Beam area, 17–18, 63, 147, 190
Beam diameter, 61–66, 197
    focusing affecting, 70
    and lateral resolution, 68
Beam profilers, 128–130, 141, 147
Bioeffects of ultrasound, 2, 132–136,
    141
    AIUM statement on, 133, 134
    mechanisms of action for, 134–135
Bistable display, 95, 147
B-mode operation. *See* Brightness-
    mode operation
Bone
    attenuation in, 23
    propagation speed in, 9
Brightness-mode (B-mode) operation,
    93–94, 99–100, 147
B scan, 94, 99, 100, 147

Calorimeters, 125–126, 141, 147
Cathode-ray tube, 93–95, 147
Cavitation, 147
    and bioeffects of ultrasound, 134,
    135
C-mode operation, 94, 101–102, 147
Compensation, 21, 84, 85, 87, 91,
    147
    measuring of, 122–123
Compression, 85, 88, 91, 147
Continuous-wave mode, 56, 61, 147
    in Doppler system, 107
Continuous-wave sound, 13, 56, 147
Conversion factors, for common units,
    192
Cosine of angle, 40, 147, 182, 183,
    190
Coupling medium, 32, 59, 148
Cross-section image, 94, 100, 102
Crossword puzzle, 144–145, 164
C scan, 94, 148
Curved reflector, 66, 70
    artifacts from, 110
cw. *See* Continuous-wave
Cycle, 148
    and frequency, 6, 7

per pulse, in imaging instruments,
    83
    and pulse duration, 13, 14
    reduction of, and longitudinal
    resolution, 50
    and spatial pulse length, 15

Damping, 50, 55–56, 58–59, 140,
    148
dB, 21, 148, 185–187
Dead zone, 148
    measuring of, 122
Demodulation, 88, 89, 91, 148
Density, 148, 171
    as acoustic variable, 5
    and impedance, 24
    and propagation speed, 8, 9, 196
    and reflection, 31, 196
    units, 190
Depth gain compensation, 85
Depth of penetration, 6, 23–24, 148
    and frequency range, 50
    units, 190
Depth resolution, 47
Disc, 148
    transducer element, 55, 61
Displacement, 148, 171
    unit conversion factors for, 192
    units, 190
Display systems, 93–105, 141
    ambiguity in, 94, 103
    A-mode, 93, 96–98, 146
    bistable, 95, 147
    B-mode, 93–94, 99–100, 147
    C-mode, 94, 101–102, 147
    gray-scale, 95, 141, 149
    M-mode, 93, 98, 150
    real-time, 72, 95, 105–106, 141,
    151
Doppler effect, 38–40, 148
Doppler shift, 40, 140, 141, 148
    detection of, 107
    units, 190
Doppler systems, 107–108
    artifacts with, 111
    continuous-wave, 107
    pulsed, 107, 108
Duty factor, 14, 140, 148
    and intensity, 19

Duty factor, *continued*
  of diagnostic instruments, 83
  units, 190
Dynamic range, 85, 88, 95, 148
  gray-scale, 95, 123
  units, 190

Echo, 45, 148
Echo-free region, 197
Effective reflecting area, 66, 148
Electrical pulse, 82, 148
Energy, 148, 172
  electrical, conversion to ultrasound
      energy, 54, 140
  in sound waves, 5
  units, 190
Enhancement, 110, 141, 148
Equations list, 167–169
Equivalent units, 191

Far field. *See* Far zone
Far zone, 62, 63, 141, 148
  beam diameter in, 63, 64, 66
Float, to measure radiation force,
    125
Focal length, 70–71, 149
Focal region, 70, 71, 149
Focus or focusing, 70–71, 141, 149
  and intensity, 17
  internal, 71
Force, 149, 170, 172
  units, 190
Fractional change in volume, 171,
    190
Frame, 105–106, 149
Frame rate, 105–106, 149
Fraunhofer zone, 63
Frequency, 5, 6, 7, 140, 149
  and attenuation, 50
  and attenuation coefficient, 22
  and bandwidth, 59
  and beam diameter, 63, 64, 66
  and depth of penetration, 23, 50
  incident, 38–40
  and longitudinal resolution, 50
  operating, 18, 56, 59, 150
  pulse repetition, 13, 56, 80, 83,
      105, 140, 151
  within pulses, 16, 59

reflected, 38–40
  and reflector roughness, 66
  resonant, 56, 152
  unit conversion factors for, 192
  units, 190
  and wavelength speed, 8, 10
Fresnel zone, 61

Gain, 85, 149, 187
  swept, 85
  units, 190
Gain compensation, 85
Gases, propagation speeds in, 9
Gating
  pulsed Doppler, 108, 149
  receiver, 94, 149
Gel, as coupling medium, 32, 59, 148
Glossary, 146–153
Gray-scale display, 95, 141, 149
Gray-scale dynamic range, 95, 123

Half-value layer or thickness, 23
Heat, 149, 172
  and bioeffects of ultrasound,134–135
  conversion of sound to, 21
  units, 190
Hertz (Hz), 6, 149, 191
Hydrophone, 124, 125, 141, 149
  as beam profiler, 130, 141

Imaging system, 80–84
  performance measurements for,
      120–123, 141
Impedance, 24, 149, 196
  of air, 59
  and reflection, 29–32, 37
  units, 190
Incidence
  normal, 29–32, 36, 140, 150, 196
  oblique, 29–30, 34–37, 140, 150,
      196
Incidence angle, 32, 34–37, 149, 196
Incident frequency, 38–40
Incident intensity, 29–31
Instrumentation, 3, 79–119
  and artifact production, 109–113,
      141
  display, 93–105, 141
  Doppler systems, 107–108, 111

208

Instrumentation, *continued*
  imaging system, 80–84
  receiver, 84–91
  testing of. *See* Performance
    measurements
Intensity, 5, 17–20, 140, 149
  attenuation of, 21, 22
  conversion from one intensity to
    another, 19
  and decibels, 185
  incident, 29–31
  of pulses, 18, 82
  reflected, 30, 35
  in sound beams, 61
  spatial considerations in, 18–20
  temporal considerations in,
    18–20
  transmitted, 30, 35
  unit conversion factors for, 192
  units, 190, 192
Intensity ratio, 23, 187
Intensity reflection coefficient, 31,
    35–36, 149, 190
Intensity transmission coefficient, 31,
    149, 190
Internal focus, 71

Joules, 191

Kilohertz (kHz), 13, 149
Kilometers per second, 8

Lateral, definition of, 149
Lateral resolution, 68–70, 141, 150
  measuring of, 122
Linear array, 72–74, 150
Liquids, propagation speeds in, 9
Logarithm (log), 150, 184–185
Longitudinal, definition of, 150
Longitudinal resolution, 15, 47–50,
    140, 150
  measuring of, 122
  and spatial pulse length, 47, 49–50,
    58–59
Longitudinal wave, 5, 150
Lungs
  attenuation in, 23
  propagation speed in, 9

Mass, 150, 171, 172, 190

Matching layer, 55, 56, 59, 150
Measurements of performance. *See*
    Performance measurements
Medium, 5, 150
  coupling, 32, 59, 148
Megahertz (MHz), 6, 150
Microprobe, 124
Microseconds, 6
Milliseconds, 13
Milliwatts, 17
Misconceptions concerning
    ultrasound, 196–197
M-mode operation. *See* Motion-mode
    operation
Motion, 171
  law of, 172
  particle, 5, 151
Motion-mode (M-mode) operation,
    93, 98, 150
Multipath, 111, 112, 141, 150
Multiple reflection, 46–47, 150. *See*
    Reverberations

Near field. *See* Near zone
Near zone, 61, 62, 150, 197
  beam diameter in, 63, 64
Near-zone length, 61–62
Newtons, 190, 191
Normal incidence, 29–32, 36, 140,
    150, 196

Oblique incidence, 29–30, 34–37,
    140, 150, 196
Oblique reflection, 34–37, 65, 66
  artifacts from, 110
Oil, as coupling medium, 32, 59, 148
100-mm test object, 121, 141
Operating frequency, 18, 150
  of pulsed-mode transducer, 56, 59

Particle, 5, 151
Particle motion, 5, 151
Penetration, depth of, 6, 23–24, 148
  and frequency range, 50
  units, 190
Performance measurements, 120–
    131, 141
  acoustic output of instruments, 120,
    124–126, 141
  AIUM 100-mm test object in, 121

Performance measurements, *continued*
  beam profile, 128–130
  imaging performance, 120–123
Period, 6, 7, 140, 151
  and pulse duration, 13–14, 56
  pulse repetition, 13,14,80,140,151
  units, 190
Phased array, 70, 72, 74, 105, 150
Photography, of displayed images, 95
Physics concepts, 170–172
Piezoelectricity, 54–55, 140, 151
Power, 17, 151, 172
  and decibels, 185–187
  units, 190
Power ratio, 85, 185–187
Pressure, 151, 170
  as acoustic variable, 5, 6
  units, 190
Probe, 55, 151
Propagation, acoustic, 2, 146, 151
Propagation speed, 6, 8–10, 140,
    151, 196
  and Doppler effect, 39
  and impedance, 24
  for pulses, 16
  and range equation, 45
  of transducer material, 56
  and transmission angle, 35–36
  units, 190
Propagation speed error, 110–111,
    141
Pulse, 151
  amplitude of, 82
  electrical, 80, 82, 148
  range of frequencies in, 59
  sound, 13, 80, 82
Pulse average intensity, 19
Pulse duration, 13, 14, 56, 80–82,
    151, 190
Pulse-echo systems, 79–83, 151
Pulse length, spatial, 15, 140, 152
  and longitudinal resolution, 47,
    49–50, 58–59
  units, 190
Pulse repetition frequency, 13, 56,
    140, 151
  and maximum depth in soft tissue,
    94–95, 103
  of pulser, 80, 83
  in real-time scanning, 105

units, 190
Pulse repetition period, 13, 14, 80,
    140, 151, 190
Pulsed ultrasound, 1, 3, 13–16,
    140–141, 151
  in Doppler system, 107, 108
  imaging system, 79–83
  transducers in, 56–59
Pulser, 80, 81, 82, 141

Quality factor (Q factor), 59, 151

Radiation force, 151
  measuring of, 125, 141
Range accuracy, measuring of, 122
Range, dynamic, 85, 88, 95, 123,
    148
Range equation, 45–46, 151
Range resolution, 47
Rayls, 24, 151, 191
Real time, 72, 105–106, 151
Real-time display, 72, 95, 105–106,
    141, 151
Receivers, 84–91, 141
Recording of displayed images, 95
Rectification of pulses, 88, 89
Reflected frequency, 38–40
Reflected sound, 1, 29–32, 34–37,
    38–40
Reflecting area, effective, 66, 148
Reflection, 1, 3, 79, 140, 151, 196
  and attenuation, 21, 41–44
  multiple, 46–47, 150
  specular, 32, 66, 152
Reflection angle, 34, 35, 151, 196
Reflection coefficient, 31, 35–36,
    41–44
Reflector, 38, 152
  curved, 66, 70, 110
  oblique, 34–37, 65, 66, 110
  roughness of, 66
  speed of, and Doppler effect,
    38–40
Refraction, 35–36, 140, 141, 152
  artifacts from, 111, 112
Registration, 152
  measuring of accuracy in, 122
Rejection, 88, 90, 91, 152
Repetition frequency. *See* Pulse
    repetition frequency

Resolution
  angular, 70
  and artifacts, 111, 113
  axial, 47
  azimuthal, 70
  depth, 47
  lateral, 68–70, 141, 150
    measuring of, 122
  longitudinal. *See* Longitudinal
    resolution
Resonant frequency, 56, 152
Reverberations, 46–47, 110, 140,
  141, 152
Risks in diagnostic ultrasound, 132,
  136–137
Roughness, reflector, 66

Safety of ultrasonic procedures, 132,
  136–137
Scan converter, 95, 141, 152
Scan lines, 105–106, 152
Scanning, 72, 152
  real-time, 72, 105–106, 141, 151
Scattering, 21, 32, 152
Schlieren system, 124–125, 130, 141,
  152
Sensitivity of imaging system, 152
  measuring of, 121–122
Shadowing, 110, 141, 152
Side lobes, 61, 141, 152
  artifacts from, 111
Sine of angle, 35, 152, 182, 183, 190
Smoothing of pulses, 88, 89
Snells's law, 35, 152, 196
Soft tissues
  attenuation in, 22–23, 41, 44
  attenuation coefficient for, 22
  beam diameters in, 63, 64
  depth of penetration in, 23, 24
  longitudinal resolution in, 49
  maximum depth in, 94–95
    in real-time imaging, 106
  near-zone length for, 61
  propagation speeds in, 9, 10, 45,
    140
Solids, propagation speeds in, 9
Sound, 5, 152
  conversion to heat, 21

properties of, 5–10
Sound beams, 61–66, 141, 152
  focusing of. *See* Focus or focusing
  unfocused, 21
Sound wave. *See* Wave, sound
Spatial average (SA) intensity, 18
  and SP/SA factor, 18
Spatial-average-temporal-average
  (SATA) intensity, 19, 20, 83
  in Doppler instrument, 108
  measurement of, 125
Spatial-average-temporal-peak
  (SATP) intensity, 19, 20
Spatial peak (SP) intensity, 18
  and SP/SA factor, 18
Spatial-peak-temporal-average
  (SPTA) intensity, 19, 20, 83
  measurement of, 125
Spatial-peak-temporal-peak (SPTP)
  intensity, 19, 20, 83
Spatial pulse length, 15, 140, 152
  and longitudinal resolution, 47,
    49–50, 58–59
  units, 190
Specular reflections, 32, 66, 152
Speed, 152, 171
  unit conversion factors for, 192
  units, 190
SP/SA factor, 18, 83, 190
Stiffness, 152, 171
  and impedance, 24
  and propagation speed, 8–9, 196
  units, 190
Strength of sound, 17, 152
Strip-chart recorder, 95
Swept gain, 85

Temperature, 153, 172, 190
  as acoustic variable, 5
  units, 190
Temporal average intensity, 19
Temporal peak intensity, 19
Testing of equipment. *See*
    Performance measurements
Thermocouple, 126, 141, 153
  as beam profiler, 130, 141
Time units, 190
Time gain compensation, 85

Transducer, 3, 13, 54–59, 140, 141, 153
  beam diameters for, 61–66, 197
  continuous-wave mode, 56, 61
  damping of, 50, 55–56, 58–59, 140, 148
  and longitudinal resolution, 59
  matching layer in, 55, 56, 59, 150
  pulsed-mode, 56–59
  single-element, 55–71
Transducer arrays, 72–74, 153
Transducer assembly, 55, 56, 153
Transducer element, 55, 153
  curved, 70
  disc, 55, 61
  thickness of, 56
Translucent region, 197
Transmission angle, 34, 35, 153, 196
Transmission coefficient, 31, 41, 43
Transmitted sound, 29, 31, 79
Transonic region, 197
Transverse resolution, 70
Trigonometry, 182–183
Tube, cathode-ray, 93–95, 147

Ultrasound, properties of, 5–28, 153
Unfocused beam, 21
Units, 189–195
  conversion factors for, 192
  equivalent, 191
  manipulation of, 189, 193–194
  prefixes for, 191

symbols for, 190
  tabulation of, 190

Variables
  acoustic, 5, 8, 17, 140, 146
  wave, 5, 153
Velocity, 8, 153, 171, 190
Videotape, of real-time displays, 95
Visualization method, 1–3
Voltage
  applied to transducer, 55, 80–82
  pressure affecting, 55
  units, 190
Voltage pulse, 56, 82, 153
Voltage pulse repetition frequency, 56
Voltage ratio, 85
Volume
  fractional change in, 171
  units, 190

Watts, 17, 191
Wave, sound, 5–10, 140, 153
  longitudinal, 5, 150
  strength of, 17, 152
Wavelength, 6, 7, 140, 153
  and beam diameter, 63
  and boundary dimensions, 32
  and frequency, 8, 10
  reduction of, and longitudinal resolution, 50
  and spatial pulse length, 15
  units, 190
Wave variables, 5, 153
Work, 153, 172, 190